About the Author

Alix Kirsta is a freelance journalist and writer. For years a professional dancer and actress, she then moved into journalism and broadcasting, and was Health and Beauty Editor of *Woman's Journal* and *Options* magazine, where she gained a reputation for exhaustive research and an interest in natural therapies. A fitness enthusiast who still works out in daily professional jazz dance classes, she takes a holistic view of beauty, seeing it as reflection of the whole body's physical and mental health.

Pg 9.

SKIN DEEP

A Top to Toe Guide to Skin Care

ALIX KIRSTA

CENTURY PUBLISHING
LONDON

TO MY MOTHER

First published in Great Britain in 1985
by Century Publishing Co. Ltd.,
Portland House,
12–13 Greek Street, London W1V 5LE

ISBN 0 7126 0922 9

Photoset by Deltatype, Ellesmere Port
Printed and bound by
Hunt Barnard Printing Ltd, Aylesbury, Bucks

Contents

Acknowledgements

Skin Deep represents the end product of a long and fascinating journey into the interior, not only of the human skin but of many other nooks and crannies of the body as well, and the book could not have been written without the advice and assistance of many eminent experts in their fields who were kind enough to spend precious time and energy answering my questions. I therefore wish to thank the renowned 'dean' of dermatology, Dr Albert Kligman, Professor of Dermatology at the University of Pennsylvania School of Medicine, for elaborating on the nature of ageing and giving both the good and the bad news with inspiring verve and vigour — and also for his stern exhortation to me to get out and stay out — of the sun! I extend thanks too to Dr Kligman's colleague Jean Ann Graham, for putting cosmetics into a totally different light, and to Dr Norman Orentreich, clinical Associate Professor of Dermatology at New York University School of Medicine, and Nancy Duir for putting on their thinking caps and magic specs and speculating on skin in AD 2000. In England I wish to acknowledge the very valuable help given to me by Dr John Gilkes for a comprehensive round up of dermatological facts from A–Z; Dr Anthony Young for analysing pigmentation disorders; Dr Rod Hay for elaborating on the habits and habitats of diverse fungi; Dr Christopher Mortimer, John Studd, and Professor Howard Jacobs for unravelling the intricacies of the hormonal system; and Dr Paul Salmon for casting light on the wonders of laser technology. Warm thanks to Rita Roberts of the Red Cross Organisation and to Len Mervyn for their unstinting support and advice; to Mary Wray at Roc for putting me on the right road to explore allergies; to Mandy Langford for revealing the extent of the influence of psyche over skin; and to Diane Miles of Vichy and chemist Michael Dinsmore for valuable nuts and bolts basic product information.

Introduction

The French, as always, have an expression for true beauty and total well-being: *'se sentir bien dans sa peau'* which, roughly translated, means to feel good, or at ease, in one's skin. Superbly succinct, it sums up that enviable state of physical-cum-emotional harmony that makes beauties of us all. The essence of the phrase conjures up to me a complexion that glows with perfect health; a face that's relaxed and radiant, free from lines and the shadows of tension, pain, stress and tiredness, defying the need for props or artifice such as thick powder, foundation, concealing creams, and other forms of cosmetic camouflage. It is further illustrated by a body whose surface contours, tautness, and silky patina reflect the fitness and healthy self-regard of its owner.

But to many women (and indeed a growing number of men) the cherished ideal of a glowing, well-behaved, near flawless skin — our so-called 'rightful heritage' — seems all too elusive a quality, and far from feeling good about, let alone *in*, their skin, its condition may elicit instead more woes and worries, physical discomfort and emotional gut feelings concerning self-image than any other aspect of the body.

Sadly, it has been my experience as a Health and Beauty Editor that while women of all ages from fifteen to seventy-five are universally concerned about the appearance and condition of their skin, the majority remain woefully ignorant about its true function and structure, its weaknesses, vulnerabilities and idio-syncrasies, and thus about what can and cannot be done to prevent or overcome flaws and disorders, improve its appearance, and guard its youth and beauty.

Certainly, whether you have a good skin is to a certain extent determined by good luck and good genes. But a third factor, good sense, places the ultimate responsibility for the state of your skin fairly and squarely into your own hands. Thus a good skin, like optimum health and fitness, can be cultivated by recognising the choices and options available for modifying the *status quo*, balancing out handicaps, improving on what nature confers, and then taking appropriate preventive or therapeutic action. Easier said than done, of course. And that's the reason for this book.

Dermatology, once the narrow province of a few specialists involved in the study of obscure and exotic skin diseases, has evolved as one of the most exciting and productive areas of medical research, and scientific advances made in this field and in complementary areas such as molecular biology, biochemistry, and high technology have contributed enormously to furthering the understanding of skin disorders.

Since skin care and dermatology are an ever-changing, vast, complex and specialised field, it's no wonder most of us are perplexed about even choosing in which direction to take our first step in negotiating that territory. There *are* secrets to having attractive, healthy, young-looking skin. Many in fact. But these have little to do with 'miracle' drugs, or with the merits of expensive skin-creams or what esoteric therapies to pursue in order to give nature the elbow. Rather, they take us into areas hitherto not often associated with the care and well-being of skin at all, realms that include psychology, hypnotherapy, the study of stress, nutrition, environmental pollution, photobiology, endocrinology, and immunology. Skin, as one endocrinologist cryptically muttered to me in the course of my research, is far too complicated a subject to be fully understood by dermatologists. I think he has a point. Good health of mind and body ultimately dictate the quality of the skin of a lifetime, as do lifestyle, occupation, and environment, putting skin where it belongs into the perspective of 'holistic' health care.

In keeping with this wide-angle, in-depth approach to skin, the ethic of prevention rather than cure is as valid as in any other area of health care. Hindsight always has perfect vision, and as with any other part of the body, most of us tend to give little thought to actively caring for or understanding the quirks and foibles of our skin, taking its condition largely for granted until problems occur. And everyone, man, woman or child, is destined to suffer a skin problem, acute or chronic, major or minor, at some time or another in their lives. It is for each one of these, and for anyone who cares about their skin that I have written *Skin Deep*.

CHAPTER 1

Skin Paradox and Profile

It is tempting to regard the skin as a mere decorative showpiece, a pretty outer wrapping which combines all the aesthetic appeal of fine silk or Sèvres with indestructability, durability and infinite adaptability as part and parcel of a lifelong guarantee. A sort of designer-made, opaque, human 'clingfilm' which, were it ever marketed synthetically, would guarantee its inventor a Nobel Prize!

With a surface appearance that ingeniously belies its hidden depths, skin is nothing if not the ultimate biological paradox. Just consider how much more it accomplishes than merely bundling up and enveloping our bones, muscles, organs, viscera and fluids while obligingly putting on an appealing front into the bargain. Few people are aware, for example, that the skin qualifies as one of the largest, most complex and hardworking organs of the body with, like every other organ, its own in-built system: three times the weight of the liver and almost as busy, constantly on the go renewing and repairing itself via an elaborate and finely synchronised self-generating mechanism.

Invisible to the naked eye, its myriad components are densely and kaleidoscopically packed together, every cell, fibre and gland representing finely tuned 'systems within a system' collectively responsible for maintaining the upkeep, health and good appearance of the finished product.

Twenty per cent fluid, ranging from just 1/50th inch thick on the eyelids to $\frac{1}{2}$ inch thick on areas such as the upper back, spread flat the skin of an average sized adult man or woman would cover roughly 3000 sq inches (1.6 sq metres) and accounts for between 6–8 lbs of total body weight.

Microscopic analysis of a square-centimetre patch of tissue

would reveal as many as a dozen or so blood vessels measuring about one yard if connected together end to end, forty-five yards of nerves with 3000 sensory cells — the 'termini' of individual nerve fibres; 200 of these specifically record pain, while twenty-five pressure receptors register tactile stimuli, two react to cold and twelve to heat. Further examination shows up the skin's principal 'workforce': 100 sweat glands and about 700 pores, a dozen hairs and hair follicles, fifteen sebaceous glands, muscles, fatty tissue, and over 3 million cells constantly renewing themselves by travelling upwards to the surface, where they die off and are shed. Since healthy skin sheds one surface layer of epidermal cells every twenty-four hours and, lizard fashion, renews itself entirely over a 21–30-day cycle, it isn't so surprising that in an average lifetime we lose as much as 40 lbs of skin particles, mainly in the form of imperceptible dust and fragments.

All Systems Go

Apart from protecting the inner tissues and skeletal structures from damage, and shaping and holding together the body with the minimum restriction, maximum stretch and resilience, the skin continuously expands and contracts, in a sense 'breathing', excreting waste matter and acting as the body's first line of defence against invasion from bacteria. There are on average 100,000 microbes per square centimetre of skin, which are impossible to remove without gravely jeopardising the skin's health since they act as a resident 'home guard', continuously attacking and destroying potentially harmful invading bacteria.

Through acting as a finely tuned thermostat, regulating body temperatures whenever the going gets too hot or too cold, skin can prove, quite literally, a lifesaver. In extremes of cold, the escape of excess body heat is prevented through immediate constriction of the surface blood vessels, while in warm or hot environments or during exercise, the capillaries expand, sending extra quantities of fresh, heated blood coursing to the surface tissues to cool off; meanwhile, the tightly coiled eccrine sweat glands pump, geyser-style, moisture out through the pores which, through evaporation, has a direct cooling effect on the body whether you're out in the desert at 120°F. or whipping up your own temperature through vigorous activity. Without this sophisticated and complex mechanism, our bodies would simply boil up and die.

Along with the kidneys, the skin is also a major organ of elimination, purifying the system and excreting up to two litres of fluid each day through its entire surface — 20 per cent of the body's total fluid loss.

Bodily dehydration can therefore have a rapid and marked effect on the appearance of the skin's outer surface, increasing the need for adequate fluid intake and the use of protective creams and lotions to prevent added surface dehydration and to guard against excessive evaporation of moisture from the epidermal tissues. Apart from moisture, adequate oxygen is also a key factor in determining the skin's overall appearance and health. While receiving nutrients essential to healthy cell activity via oxygen carried in the bloodstream to the tissues, the skin, according to some dermatologists, absorbs about 4300 litres of oxygen through its surface over a 24-hour period — 10 per cent of the intake of the lungs.

When you tot them all up, these statistics offer a lot more than a string of fascinating but superfluous information. They are, on the contrary, proof positive that the skin's performance and adaptation skills amount to those of a human machine infinitely more wondrous and awe inspiring than anything as yet dreamt up in even the most advanced examples of computer chip technology.

Where The Action Is

The form and dynamics of skin cell 'division and labour' further attest to the heterogeneous complexity of our outer envelope. Imagine a cross-section of skin as a triple layer cake or sandwich, comprising three separate yet closely interconnecting sections — gently undulating, tight-knit strata, each one vitally dependent for its function and form on the health and condition of the other two.

They are: the *hypodermis* or subcutaneous tissue at base level, whose thickness varies from person to person and from one area of the body to another and which contains basically muscle, veins and fat cells (i.e. adipose tissue).

The *dermis* or connective tissue, which is usually about 1.8 mm thick and is the chief supportive section of the surface visible skin and also dictates its strength, contour and elasticity.

The *epidermis* or skin surface, only 0.2 mm thick, which is made up of a lower basal cell layer, the epidermal 'assembly line', which produces a constant turnover of newly formed, living cells that push the preceding older ones upwards where they progressively change shape, eventually overlapping like roof-tiles or fish-scales to form a tightly impacted horny cell layer — that part of the skin visible to the naked eye — which is constantly being shed and renewed.

Thus skin is a self-propagating organ, the product of a fully automated tissue factory. Skin cells are ever 'upwardly mobile', and the surface skin we present to the world is technically speaking lifeless, like hair and nails, the finished product of a molecular and cellular assembly line whose all-round quality is ultimately determined by the synthesis of raw materials located deep within the dermis.

Not for nothing is the dermis, or connective tissue, often referred to as the 'true skin'. This springy, moist, gently undulating and pocketed infrastructure determines the bounce, bloom, elasticity and smoothness of the surface skin by providing a cushiony support system not unlike a well-sprung mattress. Basically a fibrous protein mass, the dermal tissues consist of a dense weave of collagen fibres laid down in neat parallel 'bundles' and comprising 70 per cent of the body's overall collagen content. Twenty-five per cent of all the body's protein consists of collagen, which ranks as the number one constituent of connective tissue and also acts as the matrix for bones and joints. An intricate basket-like crossweave of other protein such as reticulin and elastin — as much as 60 per cent of the body's elastin lies within the skin, determining its smoothness and elasticity — further distributes shape and tension throughout the dermis.

The gel or 'aspic' in which all these fibres lie embedded is made up of a mélange of other raw materials including hyaluronic acid, sulphuric acid, and other so-called mucopolysaccharide protein complexes which act as an intercellular 'glue' while helping to bind water within the tissues, and fibroblast cells responsible for the manufacture of collagen and, to a lesser degree, elastin. Blood vessels, nerve endings, oil and sweat glands, pores, and follicles are all situated in this halfway house in the tissues. Nutrients necessary for healthy and regular tissue synthesis are supplied to this layer via the bloodstream and interstitial (i.e. the spaces between the cells) fluids.

Dividing the dermis from the uppermost section, the epidermis, is the basal cell layer, a strip of narrow but dense activity fuelled by the nutrients that filter through from the dermis. Continuously proliferating and multiplying basal cells, intermingled with prickle cells and melanocytes, the skin's pigment-forming cells, make this the 'front line' of skin production and cell turnover. Continuously pushed upwards and slotting one on top of the other through the impetus of newer and stronger cells working their way up from below, the basal cells steadily migrate towards the skin surface, their progress marked by radical structural changes as they lose their nuclei and become elongated and narrow, i.e. 'spindleshaped'.

On their upward journey these cells also become infiltrated with keratohyalin, a granular substance secreted by the basal cell layer, which eventually turns into a hard scaly protein called keratin which presses the dead flattened cells together, interlinking and overlapping them fish-scale fashion into a tightly compressed, impacted barrier which represents the outermost, so-called 'horny layer' of the epidermis. This final metamorphosis represents the end of the line, a switchover from 'working' to 'resting' skin and the final phase in the cycle of skin production.

What prevents this top layer from assuming the leathery toughness of fingernails, horses' hooves, reptilian scales and stag's antlers, which are all made of an identical keratinous substance, is the cyclical nature of skin renewal, the imperceptible but continuous rate at which old dead cells become detached, flake off and are replaced by a new layer, preventing a build-up of hardened keratin. Any flaw or imbalance in this normally steady process of keratinisation may have a significant impact on the feel and appearance of surface skin. For example, when new cells rise to the surface too quickly and clump together, as in the case of psoriasis sufferers, the result is usually redness and scaling; the extreme dryness and cracking experienced by many elderly people is often a direct result of impaired and retarded keratinisation, coupled with extreme thinning of the skin in general. Surface skin condition is also largely dependent on the degree of moisture that remains trapped in the surface cells. For, dead as they are, these flattened interlocked horny cells remain surrounded by a thick fatty outer membrane capable of retaining moisture and so keeping the skin surface soft and pliable. The water content of all skin, excluding its underlying fatty area, ranges from 65–75 per cent, of which only 10–15 per cent is distributed within the epidermis, which explains the susceptibility of surface skin — especially as ageing reduces natural skin secretions and normal water content — to the dehydrating effects of harsh weather conditions, sunlight, central heating, air conditioning, air travel, and abrasive skin products.

Although the skin does maintain a reservoir of fluid, like any other store this is liable to depletion. Accounting for about 20 per cent of the body's daily fluid loss, up to two litres of moisture a day escapes via the epidermis, either through perspiration or, less noticeably, evaporation. Indeed the skin contains about four times more water per weight unit than muscle, so its fluid content is of fundamental importance to its softness and comfort. Evaporation of moisture is steadily replenished on those areas where oil and sweat glands are most profuse — the underarm and groin areas, feet, palms of hands, nose etc. Elsewhere, to a certain degree, in skin that is relatively young, transepidermal moisture loss is continually topped up by natural lipid secretions — a mixture of oil and water — the so-called 'acid mantle' which, because of its slightly acidic composition, also helps to repel bacteria and protect against irritation while lubricating the skin surface.

CHAPTER 2

Skin Sense and Sensibility

There is nothing that skin loves as much as ritual. Not the elaborately obsessive or ultra time-consuming variety, but the sort of simple, no-nonsense, streamlined daily regime of cleansing, moisturising and conditioning that can be incorporated into everyday grooming as effortlessly as brushing the teeth, dressing or eating breakfast. Few people are born with a truly flawless complexion, and if they are, neglect, abuse, or scant regard for the fundamentals of proper skin care soon diminishes this priceless heritage. For contrary to popular belief, perfect or top quality skin is very much a by-product of dedicated care and common sense — whereby radiant well-behaved skin becomes an incalculable return on an investment of time, insight and effort.

However it is amazing how much ignorance still surrounds the identification of individual skin types and therefore, to a certain extent, their appropriate treatment. Skin therapists, dermatologists, cosmetic surgeons and beauticians the world over still stress that the majority of women of all ages remain as woefully ignorant about the nature and needs of their skin as did their mothers and grandmothers before them, who were not given the option of learning about the skin and skin care techniques through detailed magazine articles. Perhaps the reason for today's blank spot is less a matter of Dark Age ignorance than of the conflicting theories and statements, half-baked truths, fallacies, and misleading mumbo-jumbo on the 'science' of skin care and cosmetics propagated by cosmetic manufacturers. A lot is said nowadays about how to keep skin younger, brighter, cleaner, more attractive, yet so much tendentious and misleading jargon surrounds the science of skin care that it is perhaps hardly surprising that many women either dismiss skin care as a conspiracy theory to boost the sales of expensive cosmetics, and therefore prefer to let nature take its course, or, befuddled by each new miracle product as it hits the market, use it indiscriminately or incorrectly, putting undue faith in the product itself in the hope that miracles will occur overnight.

Dermatologists as a whole scoff at the notion that skin can be compartmentalised into distinct and different 'types'. What distinguishes very dry scaly from very greasy or spotty skin they say is that certain underlying systems, i.e. sebaceous secretions and keratinisation in this case, unduly monopolise some skins thus creating problems. Doctors say it is not the skin's surface that is essentially different, but different systems within the lower strata of skin that are at play. But all this seems to be merely a matter of semantics. All that really matters to a woman, or a man for that matter, is how supple, smooth, free of blemishes, attractive to look at and well-behaved their skin is, and how best to control any quirks or foibles that may prevent it from looking and feeling its best. To begin with, individual skin type — in particular whether one's facial skin seems oily, dry, sensitive or so called normal — is only partly determined by a genetic blueprint which tends to stay with you for life, like the colour of your hair and eyes, your physical structure or timbre of voice. Skin, however, does change — often dramatically — over the years. Changes in environment and lifestyle, long-distance travel, climatic changes, diet, illness, emotional upheaval, stress, and of course the process of ageing can and will alter to a certain degree the texture, behaviour and appearance of skin and so modify either subtly or drastically its immediate needs, no matter how well defined and normally predictable its basic profile. Inconsistencies and incongruities in the appearance and behaviour of our skin tend to become less upsetting and worrying or indeed mysterious once we can acknowledge that the skin is indeed in a perpetual state of flux, due either to external or internal stimuli, physiological factors, or all three, and thus deviations or variations on our particular norm are symptomatic of skin temperament. To a certain degree, therefore, the dermatologists do have a point. Categorising skin under specific labels such as oily or dry is only partially helpful in selecting the right products and correct skin-care procedures. A certain amount of awareness and intelligent insight into the changing needs of skin is more likely to control skin that sometimes acts 'out of character' than sticking uncompromisingly to any hard and fast regimented treatment. The most successful regime is therefore one which is flexible and allows maximum adaptability within a certain framework that works for the individual with minimum fuss, to accommodate the seasonal, environmental, and physiological changing needs of human skin.

Bare Faced Truths

Broadly speaking, looking at your complexion through a magnifying mirror and studying those changes in surface texture that occur throughout an average working day will be sufficient to identify its basic type. Oily skin tends to have visible or coarse open pores, and will shine an hour or so after washing and applying makeup — sooner in a very hot environment. Overactive oil glands cause a tendency to sallowness or ashiness, spots, blackheads, while on the plus side it is less susceptible to wrinkles, lines and other signs of ageing.

Dry skin is generally fair, fine and matte, on the sensitive side, with no visible or open pores. It often feels tight after washing, chafes and flakes easily, is prone to the premature formation of fine lines and wrinkles, and is more vulnerable to the dehydrating effects of central heating, extremes of temperature and sunlight because of under-active oil glands.

Sensitive skin looks translucent and fragile, may have freckles, and is generally dry, with a tendency to become flushed, irritated and blotchy in extremes of temperature or through the use of harsh cosmetics, detergent products etc. Broken red veins, dermatitis, allergies and excessive, persistent dryness are particular problems.

Combination skin can be inherited as well as acquired over the years and generally consists of an oily coarse-grained centre 'T' panel running across the forehead and down to the chin, while the cheeks are normal or even dry. The problems of greasy and dry skin can coexist side by side.

Balanced skin is a rarity — most people over the years develop a predisposition to dryness, sensitivity or greasiness — but tends to qualify as one that is smooth textured, has invisible pores but no signs of dryness, and an even tone that is not too pale, sallow or bright. External influences and general ageing often make it err on the side of dryness.

Appearances can of course prove notoriously deceptive, and skins rarely run 100 per cent true to type. Surface symptoms may conflict disturbingly, often turning out at first glance to be not all they seem. For instance, it is perfectly possible for fine surface lines, flakiness, and blackheads to develop simultaneously if you don't clean your face regularly, spend a lot of time in a dry overheated environment, and smoke heavily. Dry skin may develop spots and tiny red bumps as a result of an unbalanced diet and scant cleansing, as well as a slow-down in the rate that surface skin cells are shed. Someone who has an inherent problem with over-active sebaceous glands can soon suffer from flakiness and dry surface lines as a result of either eating an unbalanced diet or working in an overheated office, or even by using very harsh abrasive cleansers. But using extra quantities of very rich skin cream and perhaps cleansing the skin insufficiently to prevent dryness — a common ploy used misguidedly by many women to prevent dryness — only compounds such a problem further by clogging up the follicles and preventing the free flow of sebum while allowing an accumulation of dead skin cells and general skin debris to coarsen the skin's surface, making it look dull, rough and lined. Over-zealous scrubbing with harsh antiseptic products will quite perversely aggravate oily skin, and increase oil production beneath the skin's surface through stimulating the sebaceous glands while drying out the surface of the skin — a two-in-one skin condition.

Cleansing — To Wash or Not to Wash

Cleansing is the linchpin, the absolute number one priority of any successful skin care strategy, but it is too often skimped or, worse, totally scrapped during a busy schedule, as a result of laziness, late nights and lassitude.

How exactly you decide to cleanse the face in particular remains very much a matter of personal preference. For in cleansing, as in the use of make-up, fashion dictates the medium as well as the mode. For example, to wash or not to wash? Cleansing, after all, is far from synonymous with having a good scrub with soap and water, and for every woman who claims that soap and water leave her skin feeling taut, dry and two sizes too small, there is another who swears that only a good lather makes her skin feel and look really clean. Which has cornered the secret of good cleansing? Quite simply, both, since there is absolutely no conclusive evidence to suggest that either form of cleansing scores over the other in terms either of efficiency or gentleness.

The relative merits of soap and water over cleanser and tonic have been bandied about by dermatologists and beauticians for years. If washing has of late acquired a certain primitive rough and ready image, it is only because during the sixties and seventies there was a concerted campaign on the part of cosmetic manufacturers to make us more aware of the special needs of dry, very delicate, allergy-prone skin and, consequently, cleansing lotions and creams were promoted as a soft option to the abrasive efficiency of scum lather and hard water. Today, however, as more and more women wear make-up and adopt a physically active lifestyle, there is renewed focus not only on the problems of oily or combination skin but also on the steady increase in grime and big city pollution, the pendulum has swung back the other way in favour of this most basic 2000-year-old toiletry item. Except for one significant difference. The newly promoted 'soapless soaps' and super gentle complexion bars bear little affinity, either in composition or in action, to the caustic and abrasive high alkaline products of earlier decades, and could more accurately be defined as water-soluble versions of cleansing creams. Non-alkaline, these offer all the cleansing power and wet appeal of ordinary soap combined with a smooth touch of cream cleansers, and are therefore suitable even for very sensitive skins. Complexion bars or soapless soaps are made from petroleum derivatives, don't form a scum with hard water, and shouldn't be confused with 'enriched', 'super fat', extra mild or 'baby' soaps which, contrary to the manufacturers' claims, cannot condition and moisturise the skin or alter its condition in any way, since any additives are obviously washed off with the water and thus rinsed down the drain. The same rule goes for the wide variety of antiseptic soaps formulated to control acne, spots and greasy skin conditions — any anti-bacteria or drying ingredient has only transitory and minimal contact with the skin and therefore serves no therapeutic use whatever to anyone with an oily skin. On the contrary, very strong medicated soaps may cause an allergic reaction or dermatitis, especially after repeated use.

There is, therefore, as yet no such thing as a soap which can condition or moisturise the skin. However, chemists are now working on a revolutionary new formula for a conditioning soap that sounds a contradiction in terms but could in fact improve the texture of very dry sensitive skin. Through a process called 'micro encapsulation', it is possible to trap tiny particles of oil within a lipid film which would stabilise and prevent them from washing off the face in the normal way. Should the new formula prove successful, it would herald a significant breakthrough in the synthesis of a cleanser-cum-conditioner. No matter how mild its formula, soap is always slightly alkaline; made from animal and vegetable fat, it reacts with the minerals such as calcium and magnesium salts in hard water to form a scum which can clog up and irritate the pores. The advantages of soap are of course that it removes grease and dirt on impact, cleansing skin properly, and banishing body odours caused by bacteria, sweat and grease while helping to minimise the risk of infection. Unfortunately this process not only lifts dirt, dead cells and sundry grime and oils off the skin, but also strips away its natural protective secretion — the protective 'acid mantle' which, in some people, may prove to have progressive ill effects. The skin's pH level is usually between 4.5 and 5.5, and thus slightly acidic. This factor keeps cropping up in current research into dehydration and ageing as well as skin irritation and infection, and it has been found that certain brands of make-up, cleansers, tonics and soaps, if predominantly alkaline, progressively destroy this acid barrier and eventually retard its renewal mechanism, thereby allowing the skin to become more susceptible to infection, irritation and dehydration. Research shows that it takes up to one or two hours for the skin to return to its normal acid composition after washing.

Paradoxically, very oily, acne-prone skin can react perversely to this by stepping up oil production as if to strengthen the skin's defences — a particular problem if you are trying to control an oily skin, open pores and spots through frequent washing. On the flip side of the coin, in mature or very dry skin the rate of moisture and oil secretion gets sluggish, and problems start to develop unless you use the right creams and moisturisers to help combat dryness and immediately replace the skin's buffer system by normalising its acid mantle.

For anyone totally opposed to the use of any type of soap no matter how mild, or for whom the feel of water on their face alone is anathema to good skin care, liquid or cream cleanser applied at least twice to remove every trace of make-up, dirt and natural skin secretions is a perfectly viable alternative — but only if all traces of cleanser are assiduously removed with skin tonic or freshener. Indeed, even for somebody whose skin flourishes with regular soap and water cleansing, it's vital to remember that most soaps will not dissolve make-up completely so that a liquid or cream cleanser should *first* be used to remove make-up before the face is washed. In general, the drier the skin, the thicker and oilier can be the cleanser, and usually a cleansing cream will work most effectively, while normal to oily skins respond best to a milky liquid formula which may sometimes have an added detergent substance that not only dissolves oil completely and wipes off easily with tissues or cotton wool but which, being water soluble, can be rinsed off with tepid water or skin tonic. Cleansing lotion or cream and skin tonic, or even water in the form of spring water in a spray bottle, go hand in hand — using one without the other merely creates blocked pores, blackheads, dull dingy skin, greasiness, and spots. Cleansing both morning and night should of course be second nature, though morning cleansing can be slightly more perfunctory and aimed at refreshing the skin and preparing it for make-up than the end of the day's heavy duty approach, needed to dissolve and strip away accumulated grime, perspiration, grease and stale make-up which have become deeply imbedded in the surface.

In addition to twice-daily cleansing, there are an increasing number of dermatologists and beauty therapists who recommend once or twice-weekly exfoliation or epidermabrasion using a slightly more abrasive vigorous technique to slough off dead surface skin cells, brightening, refining and softening the complexion. Exfoliation can be carried out merely by using a soft complexion brush rather like a man's shaving brush or a buffing sponge (Buff puff) made of synthetic fibre, in conjunction with a soapless soap or water-soluble cleansing cream or cleansing liquid, or else by gently loosening the surface layer of skin with a surface peeling agent. These come in a variety of forms, liquid, cream, gel, paste, in which are suspended a mass of microscopic oatmeal, almond or even plastic granules which should be massaged into the skin to lift out impurities and abrade the hardened build-up of keratin, and then rinsed or washed off. Exfoliating or peeling creams or lotions sometimes also contain a detergent ingredient and a small quantity of alcohol to supplement the cleansing action, an excellent formula for oily or very coarse-grained skin. Exfoliation should be concentrated around those parts of the face that are prone to oiliness, open pores, blackheads and coarse hardened rough skin — the chin, nose, forehead, centre of the cheeks. Never use a peeling agent around the eyes, and always apply a moisturiser or emollient cream immediately after use. One of the principal benefits of exfoliation is that it dissolves the hardened surface keratin barrier which can often make skin look dull, dry, coarse and lined, and which also prevents creams and lotions from softening the skin and improving its texture and tone. Regular exfoliation therefore helps skin creams to penetrate the newly polished exposed layer of the skin faster and more effectively, making lines and wrinkles appear less noticeable, skin texture softer and smoother. Exfoliation should be more regularly incorporated into the weekly skincare routine as the years pass, since as skin ages, its main problem is usually a gradual slowdown in the rate at which surface skin cells are shed and replaced by new skin. Epidermabrasion can help to accelerate this activity.

Masking Actions

There are few skins that don't benefit from the regular use of a face mask. Like exfoliating agents, most face masks deep cleanse and lift off accumulated dead cells, and so brighten, smooth, soften, and literally 'polish' the complexion. All leading cosmetic manufacturers include at least one mask or face pack in their skin care collections, but to find one that fits your requirements as well as your skin-type you may need to browse around a bit and read the instructions of various products. Masks fall into three main categories:

Deep cleansing masks or old-fashioned face packs which contain clays and earth, sulphur, tar and other active ingredients such as seaweed extract, may come in the form of a thick paste which hardens on the skin, absorbing grease, dirt and all surface impurities from the skin. When you rinse it off, your face is deeply cleansed, the pores temporarily tightened, and the circulation improved, giving you a healthy pink glow. Greasy and acne-prone skins can use these twice a week, normal skins once every seven or ten days: dry sensitive skins should use them only about once a month.

Moisturising and revitalising masks come in thick emollient cream form and generally contain moisturising ingredients as well as elements to stimulate the flow of blood to the skin's surface. These don't usually dry completely and you can sometimes apply them right up to the eye area — which you must not do with the other variety. The purpose of a moisturising mask is not so much to cleanse as to iron out and soften lines of tiredness and tension, improve sallow skin tone, and soften the complexion. Flower, vegetable, herbal extracts and plant oils all help to improve the skin quickly and noticeably and give a fresh and pleasant aroma. These can be used as often as desired by all skin types including those with a tendency to red veins and sensitivity.

'Quickie' refresher masks contain menthol, camphor and other cooling, astringent ingredients — often plant-based — to boost the circulation, tighten the pores, make the skin feel tingly and give it a healthy glow. They provide an excellent pep-up for tired skin, especially after a long day or before a party, but do little to cleanse or deeply condition the skin. Such masks should not be used more than once or twice a week, as they can have a drying, irritating effect.

Your Moisture Bank

At any age a moisturiser is just about the most valuable product in any one's skin-care kit. It should qualify as the one 'indispensable' you'd choose if stranded on a desert island. The smoothness and elasticity of young skin depends almost entirely on the moisture contained both in the dermis and the epidermis: if you were to take a section of human skin and allow its moisture to evaporate completely, it would resemble a wrinkled crinkly, hardened piece of chamois leather or parchment paper! In children and young girls, the skin's surface is kept supple and moist by a mixture of water and oils produced by the sebaceous glands — the normal skin secretion of a healthy skin — but this process gradually starts to slow down, showing a debit from the late twenties or early thirties onwards, and a steady evaporation of moisture sets the scene for dry, taut, flaking skin and the beginnings of fine lines and wrinkles. Skin ageing is invariably synonymous with loss of moisture; the sebaceous glands become lazy, the protective natural secretions take longer to renew, and the underlying gelatinous collagen structure hardens, losing its ability to hold water. The most obvious culprits that help deplete this moisture reservoir are sunlight, harsh cold winds, central heating, air conditioning, as well as prolonged illness, crash dieting, smoking, stress, and drinking too much alcohol.

Can we replenish moisture — given that the skin's superstructure, its keratin layer, constitutes a supposedly watertight barrier — and if so, how? Controversy remains regarding the skin's permeability. The majority of dermatologists insist that it is watertight and impermeable, although tests carried out in France over the past few years suggest that microscopic quantities of fluid can penetrate the epidermis, mainly through the hair follicles where the skin is thinnest. Dr Jean Valnet, President of the Société Français de Physiotherapie et Aromatherapie, stresses that the essential oils of plants can be traced in the urine half an hour after they have been massaged into the skin. Dr Valnet's research doesn't necessarily prove that water can get in by a similar route, but it has at least cast doubt over any hard and fast held belief that the skin absorbs nothing. So moisturisers present something of a dermatological conundrum. The only substance that makes skin soft and subtle is water, yet it is impossible, say most chemists, to introduce water into the skin. A Catch-22 situation? No longer, it would seem. Recognising that products with a high water content merely evaporate on the skin, chemists and dermatologists stress that the function of a good moisturiser therefore should be to prevent excess moisture loss from the skin.

There are two main types of moisturiser: thick water-in-oil creams and very lightweight oil-in-water emulsions or creams, which may contain up to 80 per cent water and humectants — natural moisturising substances such as urea, rosewater and glycerine, which attract particles of moisture from the air and into the skin and therefore work particularly well in warm humid atmospheres to augment the skin's own surface moisture level. Non-greasy, they are also ideal for very young skins and for those that tend to be oily and prone to spots and open pores: but a word of warning! Unfortunately moisturisers which contain very large quantities of humectant can have a perverse drying effect under certain conditions — when the weather is very hot and dry or cold and dry, or when you spend long periods in over-centrally heated or air conditioned buildings, the dry air grabs onto all that extra moisture and pulls it out of the skin. In the long run the best way to fight dehydration is with a water-in-oil cream moisturiser which is made up of a smaller percentage of water and humectant, blended with oils, fats and waxes into what is called an 'oily phase'. Oil-phased moisturisers are made in liquid or cream form. Which one you use depends mainly on how comfortable it feels on the skin, but bear in mind that the drier your skin and its environment, the richer your protective cream should be. Heavier creams give added protection in very cold weather and some extremes of temperature. Water-in-oil emulsions form an occlusive or protective barrier on the skin's surface to trap moisture and prevent it evaporating, while helping to plump out surface skin cells and make tiny lines and wrinkles less noticeable.

The terms night creams, nourishing creams, skin foods are all extremely misleading, since these are euphemisms used to describe what is basically a rich moisturising cream. The formulae are modified to give greater smoothing and softening properties, and the proportions of oils, waxes, water and other emollients varied in order to give a heavier and richer texture. Cold cream, lanolin and petroleum jelly are all examples of straightforward emollients which work to counteract dryness and irritation of the skin by softening and smoothing it and leaving an oily film to prevent evaporation of moisture from its surface. Unless your skin is very dry, there should be no need to use a so-called night cream before the age of about twenty-five; a moisturiser will provide young skin with ample protection during the night since you lose far less moisture while you are asleep than during the day. Even older women should remember that very greasy and heavy night creams tend to coarsen and clog up the pores, lead to fluid retention and puffiness, especially around the eye area, and may 'drag' the skin, possibly encouraging slackness of the tissues especially around the mouth and eyes. There are specific danger zones that you need to cosset and protect more than any other parts of your face. These are the eye area, neck and throat. Because these tissues are so fine and delicate and devoid of underlying sebaceous glands, they tend to show signs of ageing long before general skin deterioration begins. It is never too early to begin protecting these areas; fine laughter lines, dryness, crêpiness and crinkly crow's feet wrinkles can become a problem even in the early to mid-twenties — depending, as always, on how kindly you treat your skin. Too much sun bathing, screwing up the eyes, frowning, late nights, rubbing and pulling the skin around the eyes as well as applying very heavy creams and oils can all result in wear and tear. Similarly wearing rough fibres, polo neck sweaters, sun bathing, sloppy posture can make the skin on even a very young neck and chest area crepey, slack and indented with creases and 'necklace lines'. This is where neck and eye creams come to the rescue. From the twenties on, these creams are the salvation of these vulnerable parts of the face — though you may actually not be aware of this until you reach your thirties or forties. Eye creams can be worn either during the night, throughout the day, or both. Very fine lightweight creams, formulated like an oil-in-water moisturiser and disappearing instantly into the skin, are better for the day to use beneath your make-up, while richer water-in-oil emulsions provide the skin with extra lubrication and should be worn at night. A word of caution, however: never *never* overload the eyes tissues with thick greasy creams, and only apply a minute dot of cream at a time. Applying too much cream can stretch the skin, making it slack and create puffiness and bags under the eyes. If puffy eyes are a particular problem, opt for an eye gel instead of a cream to wear during the day and perhaps even during the night, especially when the weather is very warm and humid, making the eyes more likely to become puffy. Often made from gentle, deep-acting plants and herbal extracts such as camomile, eye-bright, and cornflower, these have a decongestant, firming and tightening effect on swollen slack eyelids, ironing out tiny creases and lines, and calming irritated tissue; as they leave no greasy residue, they provide a perfect, smooth, silky matte base for eye make-up during the day. Neck creams or oils on the other hand are generally made up of a richer formula because the skin on the throat, chest and neck tends to be extremely dry but rather less sensitive and delicate than the rest of the face. Creams or oils are best applied in the morning after bathing or showering and also at night, when they penetrate and nourish the skin more effectively while the neck muscles are relaxed and the skin more receptive.

CHAPTER 3
Term of Trial

Nature really seems to have it in for the very young. As if the diverse trials and tribulations of growing up compounded by the stresses of exams, early sexual or romantic encounters, and shaky self-confidence weren't enough to make the teens and the early twenties a rough passage for many an adolescent girl or boy, skin problems in the form of spots, pimples or full blown acne only serve further to pour oil — quite literally — on already turbulent waters. Neither physically harmful nor contagious, nor even a symptom of ill health, acne nevertheless rates as one of the most psychologically traumatic of skin disorders in young women and men alike. Because of the unwholesome appearance of cysts, bumps, boils, blackheads, scars and pustules — all too often mistakenly associated with lack of hygiene or an unhealthy lifestyle — it is hardly surprising that someone who is plagued with persistent serious acne rarely comes to terms with it and may develop a warped self-image and loss of confidence, a particularly devastating handicap during the emotionally vulnerable teens and early twenties. Thus the physical blight of acne is often superseded by its psychological scars since, by any standards, it ranks as a glaring antithesis to what we define as a healthy, attractive complexion.

Acne vulgaris (the term used to describe the entire gamut of pimply, greasy, skin eruptions) is seen as a prime scourge of adolescents and is most virulent between the ages of twelve and twenty odd. But to categorise it predominantly as a 'teenage disorder' is grossly to over simplify the issue, for although about 80 per cent of all teenagers *are* plagued by acne, it is by no means exclusively endemic in the very young. So-called 'teenage' acne can linger well into the twenties and thirties or worse, and may flare up in women of thirty or forty plus who have previously never suffered from spots or any other related skin problems. Acne patients, even more than those with eczema and psoriasis, make up the bulk of any dermatologist's surgery nowadays — although there is as yet no cast-iron or sure-fire preventive treatment for the condition, and doctors remain puzzled as to its precise cause. It has been estimated that a minimum of 360,000 new cases of acne are treated by doctors in Britain each year, a conservative estimate of the number inflicted, bearing in mind the countless sufferers who shun medical help and opt for over-the-counter remedies — many of them largely ineffective. One girl in every two, for example, has a persistent spot problem, and virtually all young men suffer from it, yet only one in twenty acne sufferers consult a GP or dermatologist for treatment. The disorder begins at an early age in girls, usually between the ages of twelve and fourteen, and around sixteen in boys, in whom the symptoms are usually more severe and long lasting, dragging on into the early or mid-twenties. A sense of hopelessness and ignorance of effective treatments can compound the mystery of acne and prolong its agony; it may prove notoriously persistent and impervious to the gamut of tried and tested treatments.

Despite the easy identifiable surface disfigurement, acne still remains somewhat of a dermatological enigma. Its pattern is maddeningly inconsistent, since outside the well-defined syndrome of teenage acne provoked by a burgeoning and erratic hormone production during puberty and beyond, there remains the mystery of why some young people manage to escape it altogether while others remain plagued by spots well into adulthood and even middle age. Equally mysterious is what precise hormonal adjustments commonly put a full stop to acne in the early to mid-twenties. What doctors *have* established is that acne has strong genetic links — if your mother or grandparents had it, then the chances are you will be a likely candidate sometime during puberty, especially if your skin reacts adversely to the body's production of androgens. These are the male sex hormones, principally testosterone and androsteniodone which, from puberty on, are produced in very large quantities in men and in minor amounts in women, which explains why boys usually develop more severe acne than girls.

Testosterone is the principal culprit responsible for over

activating the oil-producing glands beneath the skin, which are biggest and most profuse on the face and neck and upper back. The precise role of androgens in determining the aetiology of acne is hard to identify, but endocrinologists believe that certain men and women suffer an enzyme deficiency which permits testosterone to run riot in the body, allowing it to be converted within the skin into a by-product called dihydrotestosterone (DHT), which then over-stimulates the sebaceous glands. In women suffering from acne as well as in those who display masculine characteristics such as excess facial hair, under-developed breasts and amenorroea (a lack of periods), levels of DHT in skin tissues is 60 per cent higher than in women whose hormone levels are perfectly balanced, and it is believed that the conversion of testosterone into DHT within the skin tissue itself may well be the prime factor in precipitating the entire cycle of acne. Other possible causes for abnormally high levels of DHT in the skin are a reduction in the binding proteins (androgen binding globulin) which carries testosterone into the system, thus allowing it free access to the skin tissues, or else an inherited undue sensitivity, rather like an allergy, to testosterone. It is known, for example, that hair loss in men and some women is caused by the same abnormal sensitivity in the hair follicles to DHT.

Whether abnormally high levels of testosterone are manufactured by the ovaries and adrenal glands or are produced by the skin itself remains an intriguing question for which endocrinologists have so far only clues. Recently developed techniques for measuring the levels of hormones in skin tissue have already shown that in some women the blood draining away from the tissues carries more hormones than that entering the tissues, which implies that the cells themselves are prime offenders in the manufacture of testosterone. The target of this hormonal imbalance, whatever its origins, in acne sufferers is the pilo-sebaceous unit — the hair follicle or pore duct with its underlying normally well-behaved oil-producing gland. In acne sufferers this area becomes the site of two mutually antagonistic processes — increased oil secretions coupled with accelerated cell production (hyperkeratinisation) within the basal and epithelial cells lining the follicle. It is this secondary cell activity which, even more than the extra secretion of oils, accounts for the worst features of acne. Without hyperkeratinisation, over-active oil glands will merely give a man or a woman a greasy but clear and unblemished skin. Hyperkeratinisation, however, seems to account for the formation of spots and pimples. In normal healthy skin, cells are shed freely and regularly, but in acne sufferers, who are thought to suffer a genetic defect which makes sebum secretions stickier, more copious and liable to adhere to the follicle walls, the cells become increasingly tackier and clump together more readily without ever sloughing off properly, with the result that the pores become sludged up with dead cells, debris and surface oil secretion. To make matters worse, the free flow of sebum is suppressed and dammed up altogether by this barrier of thickened cells, narrowing the follicle and making the oil glands swell up and eventually leak into the adjacent tissues, producing those familiar painful bumps, red swellings, cysts and infected abesses. Less unsightly but often just as resistant to treatment are the blackheads, whiteheads, small closed comedones and pimples which result from comparatively super-ficial pore blockage. Another contributory factor to the scenario of acne is the abnormal inflammatory reaction of the skin to these blocked ducts. The normal skin bacteria break down the accumu-lated sebum into irritating 'free fatty acids', which explains the most distressing aspect of the condition — redness, swelling, unsightly cysts and pustules. For example, studies show that injections of these fatty acids into healthy skin tissue will inevitably result in the formation of acne. Increasing numbers of skin specialists now believe that severe cystic acne erupts as a result of an abnormal sensitivity of the skin's white defence cells to the build-up of excess sebum, so that acne in a sense is rather like having an in-built allergic response to one's own skin secretions. Proponents of this 'micro environment' theory of acne believe that further research into the different types of bacteria produced in the follicles as well as the composition of sebaceous secretions in acne sufferers may well explain the pathological difference between normal and acne-prone skin.

Cause and Effect

The acne syndrome therefore seems based on a clear chain of events, although what remains puzzling is why the symptoms sometimes linger well past puberty and adolescence when hormonal flux which characterises the onslaught of sexual maturity has in fact stabilised, or why 5 per cent of women sufferers may continue to suffer severe acne into their late twenties and thirties. Doctors emphasise that inflammation of normal skin bacteria can be aggravated through excessive humidity, working in garages, or with machinery that uses up certain oils, taking medicines such as bromides, cough medicines, antiepileptic drugs, using certain cosmetics, premenstrual hormonal fluctuation, taking the Pill (especially the new low-oestrogen, high-progesterone or progesterone-only brand), insufficient sleep, general stress or emotional trauma, which can upset the finely tuned pituitary gland responsible for governing the clockwork precision with which hormone levels are maintained. American studies suggest, for example, that acne is significantly aggravated in young people during the exam periods.

Many familiar myths regarding acne are, however, rapidly being shot down. Diet, for instance, is believed to have little effect on chronic acne, though eating too many fatty or sweet foods, iodides, bromides or androgenic substances including corn oil, peanut oil and wheatgerm oil which raise the body's testosterone and/or DHT levels, can certainly cause someone with otherwise perfect skin to develop the odd crop of spots. Dr James Fulton, a research scientist with America's Acne Research Foundation, believes iodine (as used, for instance, in vitamin pills) can induce acne, irritating acne-prone skin. Iodine irritates the skin as it is excreted through the sebaceous glands. Dr Fulton therefore advises acne sufferers to avoid kelp, sea salt, asparagus, broccoli, iodised salt, wheatgerm, and shellfish. Nor will 'settling down and having a baby' — that unrealistic panacea prescribed by well-intentioned GPs of an earlier generation — have much effect on chronic acne. On the contrary, spots and greasy skin disorders can flare up after childbirth, as they do sometimes when a woman comes off the Pill, due to a sudden drop in hormone levels. Neither is sunlight the all-healing influence it is often made out to be. Although spots and greasy skin conditions may at first improve in the sun because of its drying effect, the skin surface very soon becomes thicker to protect itself against burning, and the follicles can become blocked, suppressing the flow of sebum and setting off an even more severe cycle of ultraviolet, light-induced greasiness and acne. Contrary to popular belief, rarely does insufficient cleansing exacerbate acne, in fact rather the opposite. Fierce scrubbing with abrasive lotions, detergents and harsh caustic soaps can traumatise the skin, toughening up its surface — just like sunlight — and further sealing off the offending blocked pores with a plug of hardened keratin. What is more, vigorous scrubbing can also give a fillip to sebum production, compounding the vicious circle even further. Nevertheless the paramount commandment to all acne sufferers still stands — never ever ever pick or squeeze the spots! Self-control, or its lack, can make a phenomenal difference both in the development and surface spread of acne as well as in the future healing processes deep within the damaged collagen infrastructures. Often carried out in desperation, a mixture of self-hate and misery, or possibly all three, trying to 'doctor' any type of eruption can only lead to cross infection and gross exacerbation of the existing problem. In more serious cases of large pustules and cysts and bumps, squeezing creates sheer mayhem, pushing inflammation and infection deeper into the skin and leading to permanently damaged tissue, chronic inflammation and most distressing of all, deep pitting and scarring, a legacy of a lifetime since acne scars are notoriously hard to eradicate or fade even with surgical procedures.

But despite the grim surface picture, today's acne sufferers have a lot more to smile about than their counterparts of an earlier generation. In all but the most stubborn and seriously disfiguring cases, specialists favour localised external treatment rather than the prescription of strong systemic drugs which alter the physiological pattern of acne but at the cost of drastic side-effects. The milder types of acne, sporadic outbreaks of blackheads, whiteheads, and small surface spots with relatively little redness or swelling can often be cleared up with patience and perseverance by using a drying agent such as sulphur, resorcinol, or one of the newer more powerful benzoyl peroxide or ethyllactate lotions designed to dissolve the obstructing keratin plug within the follicle by drying, peeling away and so eliminating dead skin cells. Topex, Oxy 5 or 10, Acne Gel, and Quinoderm are just some popular and effective over-the-counter keratolytics which contain benzoyl peroxide; another, TRI-AC, contains ethyllactate. Because they clear up blocked pores and greasiness by initially irritating the skin to cause dryness and peeling, some skins may experience an adverse reaction, but this is very temporary and treatment can be discontinued if it becomes too severe. Regular use of a mild medicated facial wash such as Biactol, Swiss Bio-

Facial, Clearasil, or Clear Guard helps to control surface accumulation of grease but has no effect on the condition itself, since the offending bacteria that perpetuate acne lie within the follicle not outside it. In more severe cases of comedonal or infected pustular acne, a more powerful keratolytic or skin peeling agent called retinoic acid (Retina A), a synthetic vitamin A-derivative, may be prescribed for topical application where it also works by irritating and drying out the affected areas, allowing the dry plugs of grease and cell debris to be lifted out of the ducts and preventing the obstruction of oil. One over-the-counter product Monclerderma contains a group of chemicals similar in structure to vitamin A which unplug blocked pores and control spots with rather less drying and irritating side-effects than Retina A or even commercial products containing benzoyl peroxide.

Alternatively a dermatologist may inject larger lesions and cysts with cortisone. Tremendous controversy now surrounds the use of corticosteroid ointments (Betnovate, Synalar, etc.) for skin complaints such as acne. Although these often provide highly effective and fast relief from inflammation and irritation, they are now known to possess a rebound effect — once use is stopped, especially after a long period, the condition may return, often flaring up more seriously than before. The skin therefore is 'hooked'. Dermatological side-effects moreover can include thinning and atrophy of the skin, increased hair growth, red veins, and depigmentation.

Softly Softly

Many doctors still prefer to adopt a softly softly approach when treating acne, reserving very hard line invasive treatments or the use of powerful drugs only for those cases which have failed to respond to gentler methods. Of these, the very unsightly 'blazing' acne marked by redness, discomfort and swelling beneath the skin, as well as severe surface infection, presents one of the greatest challenges to dermatologists. Large cysts can either be incised and drained or else frozen with a carbon dioxide liquid snow 'slush' which initially sets off a massive inflammatory reaction that subsides as the cyst dries out. In other rare and stubborn cases large cysts can be directly injected with a steroid solution to control and prevent any further inflammation of the skin. The use of antibiotics to treat acute acne has also come in for its fair share of controversy. Although drugs such as tetracycline, septrin or minocin should only be prescribed when all else appears to have failed to control stubborn bacteria and oil production, and even though the doses are relatively small (usually 2×50 mg tablets daily) because it is prescribed for periods of between six weeks to three or six months, side-effects are the same as with any antibiotic therapy. These may include digestive upsets, depression, nausea, vaginal thrush, over-sensitivity to sunlight and even worsening of the skin condition once treatment is stopped. Tetracycline and other antibiotics also cannot be given to pregnant women or those not on effective contraception as it can damage the unborn fetus. However, as one professor of dermatology said recently, if the dosage and timing of antibiotic therapy are carefully monitored to suit individual patients, chronic acne can often respond spectacularly without any undue side-effects. The skin cannot get hooked if therapy is phased out gradually to avoid a rebound action and this must also be done at the right time of year — for instance in winter, when the oil glands are less highly geared to action — in exactly the same way that one would balance and reset a thermostat. The guiding maxim is therefore discretion and a gentle touch.

Meanwhile other powerful drugs are being tested successfully in the battle against very long-term, persistent acne. Diane is the brand name of a new hormone treatment based on a chemical called cyproterone-acetate which blocks the action of male hormones in the body. Because it causes menstrual irregularities, it has been balanced with the female hormone oestrogen to give 100 per cent effective contraceptive effect. Also used for excessive body hair, treatment consists of taking a three-week-calendar pack of tablets with one pill-free week to induce withdrawal bleeding. Because of its relatively high oestrogen content — 50 microgrammes per tablet — this particular treatment is obviously unsuitable for women over thirty or those who cannot take the Pill. It is for obvious reasons, because of its feminising effects, a no-go treatment for male sufferers. Launched just a few years ago, Diane has a poor track record in treating severe acne mainly, say some specialists, because its anti-androgen levels are too low, at 2 millogrammes, to have any significant or lasting effect. Its 50 microgramme content of oestrogen, in the light of current findings about the links between high-dose contraceptive pills and the risk of thrombosis and heart attacks, makes this in any case a highly dubious form of acne therapy, and it is not favoured by most leading endocrinologists. Originally devised to treat baldness and hirsutism in women, standard systemic anti-androgen based on doses of up to 50 millogrammes of cyproterone-acetate, balanced with a lower oestogen content, if carefully prescribed, can over a period of one to two years control even extremely virulent female acne with minimal side-effects, of which tiredness is the commonest symptom. Diminished libido and an impaired sperm count are, however, common side-effects that preclude systemic anti-androgen treatment for men.

Certain specialists report good and rapid results in treating acne in both men and women with an anti-androgen solution applied to the skin's surface; interestingly enough, the testosterone-inhibiting compound does not appear to be absorbed systemically, therefore male patients suffer none of the de-masculising effects inherent in systemic therapy.

Given that about 90 per cent of acne sufferers of both sexes who seek medical treatment do respond, albeit in varying degrees, to antibiotic therapy, there remains a 10 per cent hard core of incurables, those who simply don't respond well or who have a very quick relapse when therapy is stopped. Not normally given to hyperbole, the staid medical journal *The Lancet*, when reporting on a new treatment a few years ago, said 'It scarcely seems credible but after centuries of medieval and sometimes messy darkness, acne sufferers may be glimpsing a new and genuine dawn.' The cause of this enthusiasm is a drug called 13-Cis retinoic acid (or isotretinoin), marketed by Roche under the tradename Roaccutane, a powerful synthetic vitamin A-derivative and one of a large group of oral retinoids that are proving highly successful in the treatment of numerous skin disorders. Taken orally, Roaccutane seems to provide very significant long-term remission in acne patients once dismissed as beyond help. Originally developed as a possible cure and prevention of cancerous and pre-cancerous skin lesions, retinoids appear to work by altering the ecology and 'mechanism' of the skin, inhibiting the over-production of surface skin cells, reducing oil secretion, and also affecting inflammation and immune responses. Double blind clinical studies carried out recently at Leeds General Infirmary under the auspices of one of Britain's leading acne specialists, Dr William Cunliffe, have shown that over 90 per cent of patients with severe acne that had previously proven unresponsive to long-term antiobiotic therapy reacted dramatic-ally to isotretinoin. The most encouraging aspect of this latest treatment — only prescribed as a last resort for very serious cases — is that remission is prolonged, up to three or five years in some cases, with a very low incidence of relapse after a standard sixteen-week treatment course. Isotrentoin seems to break the cycle of abnormal processes which initiate and perpetuate acne, primarily by drastically cutting down sebum production, altering the chemical composition of skin secretions, and shrinking the swollen and distended sebaceous glands, while also inhibiting keratinisation, unplugging blocked follicles and soothing in-flammation. A potent drug, it is not without certain side-effects including dryness and mild itching of all the membranes — the lining of the mouth, eyes, and nasal passages — chafing of the lips, nose bleeds, and muscle and joint ache, especially in people who are physically active. The drug also elevates the level of blood fats including cholesterol, so treatment must be strictly supervised and includes regular liver function tests. Animal studies show that retinoids can cause foetal damage, so women must take very strict contraceptive measures to ensure that they do not get pregnant during or up to one year after therapy.

Somewhere between heart-breaking chronic acne and sporadic minor flare ups of spots and pimples hardly worth mentioning, there is the 'middle of the road' problem skin which is neither disfiguring enough to merit medical attention nor fully respon-sive to home treatments. It is in this amorphous grey area that a good therapist or beautician can still offer the best chances of cultivating clear skin. Therapists treat both mild and severe pimples and blackheads and acne problems by steaming and extracting whiteheads and/or blackheads and the use of sulphur masks as well as special superficial or deeper peeling techniques to help refine the surface skin, clear out the follicles, and improve scarring. Other therapists practise American-style megavitamin therapy to treat many types of skin disorders; acne sufferers may be prescribed mega doses of synthetic vitamin A (in doses of over 25,000 international units, natural sources of A can affect the liver, causing fatty deposits) and zinc. This combination helps to diminish over-activity of the sebaceous glands, eventually cor-recting excessively greasy skin and hair and healing infection and inflammation. Clay has been used since the year dot to treat skin complaints including acne with success, and some therapists prescribe clay treatment to be taken in large pellet form doses for internal use and poultice applications to drain out skin impurities and promote rapid healing of inflamed tissues.

CHAPTER 4

Prime Time

If there is any optimum golden age of skin, any period that reflects a woman's best years by the glow and good behaviour of her complexion, it is surely the period from around twenty-five to forty or forty-five, when the turmoil of the teens with its concomitant skin problems abates and the degenerative changes of the menopause and natural ageing processes are still far ahead.

Golden age or no, a radiant, stable, trouble-free skin is nevertheless dependent on hormonal equilibrium, and skin temperament will still be dictated — albeit less dramatically than at puberty — by the hormonal flux and flow that marks a woman's reproductive life-span. And how fraught with ups and downs and idiosyncrasies these fertile years often prove to be for many women, encompassing ovulation, menstruation and its attendant pre-menstrual syndrome, conception, contraception, pregnancy, childbirth, lactation, and the onset of the menopause either as a natural phenomenon or artificially — sometimes prematurely — induced through partial or total hysterectomy. Each of these events from the monthly 'curse' to childbirth represents a major or minor landmark in a woman's biological destiny and one that to a lesser or greater degree, noticeably or imperceptibly, affects and alters her well-being through fluctuating hormone production, which in turn implicates other bodily biochemical and biological changes and therefore may be reflected by the behaviour and appearance of the skin.

The Pill

The days when dermatologists prescribed the old-fashioned high-dose oestrogen pill to alleviate spots and pimples have passed with the advent of the safer low-dose oestrogen/pro-gestogen or progestogen-only 'mini pill'. Apart from its obvious risks and side-effects, the Pill as an acne cure was never all that it was trumped up to be in the first place. Effective only in controlling sebaceous activity if its oestrogen content hovered around 40–50 microgrammes — a dose recognised today as unacceptably high and fraught with risk factors for women of any age — acne often rebounded in a more virulent form whenever a woman stopped taking the Pill as a form of therapy. Today's low-dose Pills have virtually no impact on spots and acne. Indeed, rather the opposite. Increased levels of progestogen, whose chemical structure has an affinity with the male sex hormone testosterone, can cause spots in certain women with over-active sebaceous glands or those with a marked sensitivity to testosterone. Experimenting with different brands of the contraceptive pill may, however, solve the problem. Some women can also develop a temporary breakout of post-pill acne when coming off it, due to the subsequent resurgence of previously repressed hormone production. However, such problems tend to diminish greatly as a woman reaches her mid to late-twenties or thirties.

Far more common than pill-induced acne is the skin photosensitivity and hyper pigmentation suffered by many women on the Pill who go into the sun. Dull, dark, muddy, brown-looking blotches can appear, mainly on the face and in particular on the upper lip — giving a moustache-like effect — the forehead, and around the lower eye socket. Also a phenomenon of pregnancy, chloasma, or the so-called 'mask of pregnancy' can develop gradually, beginning with very small patches dotted here and there, and is extremely stubborn to remove once developed. Its precise cause is unknown, but it is believed that, as in pregnancy, the Pill, which mimics the hormonal changes that occur in pregnany (it works after all by fooling a woman's body into believing that she is already pregnant, so that no further pregnancy can occur) causes increased and irregular production of melanocytes which develop under the stimulus of ultraviolet light. Chloasma can occur just as easily under a sunbed as in strong natural sunlight, and once the condition has developed it can only be treated with a bleaching cream to even out the dark patches. Treatment must be long-term and persistent, as even then the evening-out process may prove incomplete or patchy.

*Eat Yogurt when on
Antibiotic)*

Wearing a total sunscreen to prevent the skin from turning brown is the most dependable way of preventing the development of brown patches from occurring in the first place. Hyper-pigmentated patches, alas, never fade, even when the skin's overall tan disappears, and the blotchiness is prone to linger through the winter months, casting greyish-beige shadows over parts of the complexion. Camouflage is therefore the best bet in this case to lighten the areas of darker skin tone.

By altering the normal, slightly acidic ecological balance of the vagina, long-term use of the contraceptive pill can cause thrush, a yeast infection usually accompanied by a white curd-like discharge and/or itching and soreness of the vagina and the skin of the outer area. Taking plenty of B-complex vitamins in the form of whole grains, live yoghurt, skimmed milk, and green leafy vegetables can help to counteract alkalinity of the vagina — doctors often suggest eating yoghurt daily when taking anti-biotics for the same reason that these destroy the body's beneficial protective bacteria as well as those that cause infection and inflammation, thereby setting the scene for a yeast infection. If allowed to go untreated, thrush may spread further to cause a nasty form of redness and itching called anogenital prurigo. An intensely irritating skin condition, this can make life almost intolerable for most women, and the fastest and most effective treatment is the localised application of a nystatin cream or nizoral tablets taken internally to bring the infection under control. Vulval and perineal viral warts are known to grow at a terrific rate and often to a very large size during pregnancy, and women on the Pill may also develop similar problems which can be treated with the local application of a special podophyllin-based tincture.

Pre-menstrual Syndrome (PMT)

Regular or intermittent outbreaks of spots, cysts and acne blemishes are a common, if relatively minor, feature of PMT and generally occur around the time of ovulation, fourteen days before a period is due, or else just prior to or in conjunction with menstruation. Exactly why the skin erupts at this stage is something of a mystery, as indeed is the entire conundrum of PMT which, according to Senior Consultant Gynaecologist at Kings College Hospital, John Stud, may be due to just about every and any hormonal imbalance in the book and not to any single cause such as the currently fashionable theory of progesterone deficiency. It is, however, possible that in the last fourteen days of the cycle, diminishing levels of oestrogen, possibly offset by relatively high levels of progesterone, allow the sebaceous glands to pump out extra quantities of sebum. Sore, sensitive breasts and puffy dimpled tissues due to fluid retention — one of the commonest pre-menstrual disorders — can be triggered by any number of factors as diverse as elevated oestrogen levels, very low progesterone, very high progesterone. Over-production of prolactin, secreted in high levels in women who breast feed their babies and the hormone implicated in infertility, as well as excess production of another hormone, aldosterone, are also believed to be possible culprits in PMT in certain women. Any of these, or a combination of these factors, can cause the body to retain salt and tissue to become fluid-logged — a contributory factor incidently in outbreaks of PMT-linked acne. Diuretics which cause loss of water can be highly effective in reducing the puffiness, discomfort and even flare-ups of the skin that accompany excess fluid in the body, but in some cases side effects include weakness, drowsiness, lethargy, and muscle cramps due to loss of salt as well as potassium. Diuretics can also increase the skin's sensitivity to sunlight causing rashes, redness, itchiness and blotchiness. If excess potassium, which along with sodium helps to regulate the water balance of the body, is also flushed out as a result of taking diuretics, then this in itself can encourage a rise in salt levels and cause further fluid retention. Eating potassium-rich foods such as bananas, apricots, and dates, and drinking fresh fruit juices whose mineral content is rapidly absorbed by the body is a safe, simple and highly effective way of maintaining a correct sodium/potassium ratio and may be sufficient to combat pre-menstrual fluid retention altogether.

Vitamin B6 deficiency, a common side-effect is some women taking the Pill, has also been implicated as a contributory cause of PMT and is another current pet theory that has been the subject of considerable medical research over the past few years. Doctors at the Pre-menstrual Syndrome Clinic at St Thomas's Hospital report that a number of PMT symptoms, including fluid retention, appear to respond well to a supplementary B6 therapy sometimes taken in conjunction with oil of evening primrose (the two seem to work synergistically) a week or two before menstruation.

Dieting

Obsession with self-image, especially weight, body size and shape — usually governed by criteria established by the media as the self-styled arbiters of fashion and sexual attractiveness — is, from the teens until well into the middle and menopausal years, often inextricably related to a woman's self-confidence and esteem. The shape she perceives in the mirror each day, for better or worse, fashions her sense of personal worth and desirability, an image that can often, as in the case of those suffering anorexia nervosa, become totally distorted, leading to compulsive neurotic dieting to the point of self-denial and malnutrition.

The quest for physical perfection, along with that other chimera, everlasting youth, accounts for the yearly burgeoning billion-pound industry in diet and slimming books, slimming magazines, diet aids, exercise classes, and figure-shaping treatments, and as such, accounts even in the most well-adjusted and intelligent of women for blinding loss of reason in the name of weight loss. Weight loss, however, can carry with it the very real risk of an accompanying diminution of well-being since, when it comes to rigorous crash dieting, the end almost invariably *never* justifies the means. For loss of stamina, strength, physical health as well as a deterioration in looks and in particular skin condition, is more often than not the net gain of very rapid and extreme loss of weight. Prolonged periods of stringent dieting or up and down yo-yo weight changes, eating a very restricted faddy diet or worse, little or no food at all as in the case of anorexia, whilst having no lasting effect on weight or physical shape in the first place can, on the other hand, leave permanently damaging and devastating scars on body skin, connective tissue and facial contours. In anorexics, for example, the impact on fertility — severely depressed hormonal production, amenorroea (absence of periods) — causes changes in bone and skin tissue akin to those suffered by women with severe symptoms of oestrogen deprivation during the menopause, causing the skin eventually to become severely dehydrated, atrophied, and thin to the point of translucency. One of the earliest forms of skin damage, though not nearly as invidious as that triggered by anorexia, occurs during the teenage years or even earlier when boys as well as girls, usually due to an unhealthy diet rich in sweets and fatty foods, become chronically obese, developing stretch marks on the stomach, buttocks, hips, thighs, upper arms, and breasts where the skin has quite simply become stretched beyond its natural capacity to give. When this excess weight is eventually shed these stretch marks remain, though they tend to fade from livid red to a pale silvery grey and the skin, with youthful resilience, usually springs back into shape again without becoming slack or creased.

However, although the degree of skin extensibility — the rate at which when pinched, it snaps back into place again — is genetically predetermined, it is also very much a prerogative of youth which begins to diminish imperceptibly from the late twenties onwards, often accelerated by such factors as diet, illness, and the use of medicines and drugs. Therefore, very dramatic weight gain followed by extreme weight loss after the age of thirty or so, when the skin's structure is already beginning to weaken and is less able to contract back and give a snug fit once over-stretched, can all too easily rupture the elastin fibres in the dermis, the rubber band network which gives the skin its tautness and firm contour. Thus a legacy of slack, sagging, crêpey, creased skin, and rolls and folds of surplus skin and flesh await the obsessive dieter as well as those who allow themselves to become chronically obese in the first place. Pendulous or distended and atrophied breast tissues, a tummy lined concertina-style, dimpled pitted skin on thighs and buttocks are just some of the trademarks of an ill-fitting epidermal uniform that has become a size too large for its owner, no longer wrapping neatly around the underlying contours.

Sadder and more immediately evident still are the facial changes that occur as a result of frequent and rigorous dieting. It is one of life's more exasperating axioms that the face, unlike the body, wears extra weight rather well, looking firmer, younger, less stretched and strained when plumped out with an underlying layer of adipose tissue to act as an age and stress 'buffer', plumping out creases, tiredness and expression lines which tend to become more readily etched on to a lean or bony face. If only we could gain or lose weight selectively! Losing even just a stone or so in weight is alas inevitably imprinted to a degree on the facial contours and neck, leading either to a gaunt, tired and 'drawn' look or worse, to a crêpey skin and droopy expression, with the appearance of folds and creases on the neck and sides of the mouth and nose, a hollowing of the cheeks more gaunt than glamorous, and a blurring and slackness around the jaw line, all of which can add years to a man or woman's true age.

What's more, following an unbalanced diet can cause dehydration and sallowness of the skin as well as a dull, muddy, lacklustre complexion, especially if protein and vitamins A,C,B-complex are severely restricted. Appetite suppressants such as amphetamines, powerful diuretics and other potent diet drugs sometimes prescribed by unscrupulous practictioners at slimming clinics can not only wreak havoc with the function of the vital internal organs and seriously affect bodily functions, but may do untold damage by depleting the body of essential nutrients, setting its glandular activity haywire; this in turn may open up a self-perpetuating syndrome of indirectly and directly related skin, hair and nail disorders. Short-term fasting or eating a mainly alkaline diet of salad, raw vegetables, fruit and fresh fruit juices for anything from three to ten days can, on the other hand, work wonders in detoxifying the system, counteracting acidity, purifying the bloodstream, and allowing the body to rest and repair itself, thereby making the skin look clearer and brighter, its texture more refined, radiant and less prone to blemishes. These changes are all the more marked if a purifying diet follows a prolonged eating binge or a massive intake of very sweet, spicy, rich and fatty foods.

Pregnancy

Women who are pregnant are often described as being at their most beautiful, their skin radiant, smooth and well behaved. Cliché it may be, but an eminent obstetrician agrees that pregnancy 'is the best thing that can happen to the skin because the body produces levels of oestrogen far in excess of those that could safely be administered in pill form'. Since oestrogen is the beneficial hormone that confers suppleness, moisture, smoothness and other useful attributes on the skin from adolescence to the menopause — and beyond depending on how lucky you are — it is hardly surprising that many skin problems including acne, excess greasiness or dryness are reversed, or reduced, and erratic skin behaviour often stabilised for good. But of all the upheavals and readjustments that a woman's body experiences during her fertile years none are more profound or cataclysmic than those accompanying pregnancy and the immediate post-natal period. Therefore there are certain exceptions to the 'bloom of woman-hood' theory. Some women may develop skin irritation on isolated areas of the body or an itchy red rash called intertrigo, which usually occurs beneath the breasts and in the groin and is more common in those who are overweight, perspire profusely, or tend to be lax about personal hygiene. The skin first becomes moist, then sore and inflamed, and eventually covered in a reddened, scaly, irritating rash. Frequent bathing and the use of talcum powder or calamine lotion helps to treat the condition, while making sure not to gain too much weight can, as in the case with haemorrhoids, often prevent it occurring altogether.

Skin irritation takes on very definite markings during pregnancy and is usually deeper and more pronounced in women with dark hair than those with fair or red hair. At about the fourteenth week the nipples and areola, the dark pink surrounding area, become increasingly pigmented, the darker tone sometimes spreading outside the areola onto the pale breast tissue itself. Any dryness of the nipples can be prevented by using a bland lanolin-based cream to condition the tissues. Women with flat or inverted nipples for whom future breast feeding may therefore prove a problem can 'tease out' their shape both by manipulation — moulding and drawing out the area between the thumb and index finger — and with the help of breast shells worn underneath a brassiere so that the nipple protrudes through the aperture onto the flat surface of one side of the shell. The shells must only be worn as long as they feel comfortable, as the skin around the nipple can easily become sore and tender. The time to begin wearing breast shells depends largely on the degree of inversion of the nipple, although most specialists advocate wearing them during the last six to eight weeks of pregnancy, initially for one or two hours a day and then for progressively longer periods each day until after three or four weeks they can be comfortably worn throughout the day.

At fourteen weeks into pregnancy the stomach characteristically develops a *linea nehra*, a dark line which runs from the umbilicus straight down to the pubis. Like the pigmentation of breast tissue outside the nipple and areola, the line fades gradually over a period of months following childbirth. Facial pigmentation, often a greater source of irritation and self-consciousness than bodily markings, occurs in late pregnancy and resembles the muddy blotchiness some women develop when sunbathing while taking the Pill. Sometimes described as the butterfly mask of pregnancy because of its butterfly-shaped configuration, the outline covers the cheeks and becomes more noticeable as a result of exposure to the sun. Although facial pigmentation does tend eventually to fade after childbirth, the more the skin has been exposed to sunlight, the more stubborn and persistent these patches can be and the more likely they are to intensify during subsequent tanning sessions. Use of a hydroquinone bleaching cream can help to minimise and even entirely remove the offending blotches, but the results more often than not may turn out mottled and uneven, with the added danger that the surrounding skin may become bleached by mistake, making the darker parts and the demarcation line appear more noticeable.

To the majority of women the greatest single bogey and distressing aesthetic price that must be paid during pregnancy — and forever after — is the formation of stretch marks. Unscrupulous beauticians have coined a small fortune by exploiting women's self-consciousness and unhappiness over these scars by promoting a panoply of so-called 'regenerative' treatments, miracle serums, oils and creams, and massage techniques purportedly capable of fading stretch marks or removing them altogether. But the harsh truth of the matter is that once the skin fibres and cutaneous tissues have been ruptured, causing stretch marks, they can *never* be removed or even very greatly improved. In most cases not even cosmetic surgery can eliminate them, since all that a surgeon can do is to tighten slack tissues which remain marked or striped — he cannot replace flesh whose surface is already scarred. Based largely on misleading, tendentious humbug, commercial cosmetic treatments to eliminate scars should be dismissed with all the contempt and scepticism that they merit.

In many cases time will, however, tone down the livid bright tones and raw appearance of stretch marks, and as these fade, so the scars become more silvery and less pronounced and therefore less distressing. Whether a woman will get them at all or how extensive and pronounced they turn out to be is totally a matter for conjecture, and it depends to a certain degree on the amount of hormones, progesterone in particular, that circulate in the body during pregnancy. High hormone levels predispose to fluid retention and also, by helping to convert calories into fat, cause the body to lay down extra layers of fatty padding, thus accounting for a very rapid increase in weight. While there is absolutely nothing that can be done to regulate hormone production during pregnancy, tremendous control *can* and *should* be exerted over the amount of food eaten and the extent of weight gained over the entire nine-month period. Not only do such widely bandied about (and downright unhealthy) platitudes as the 'need to eat for two' not have any scientific validity, but they increase a woman's risk of developing haemorrhoids, constipation, varicose veins, diabetes, high blood pressure, and swollen legs as well as stretch marks as a result of gaining too much surplus weight — which, incidently, is *not* automatically shed after the baby is born.

Controlling weight gain as much as possible while eating a healthy, well-balanced diet is the simplest and surest policy of preventing the scars of pregnancy. Taking extra care of the skin on breasts, tummy, hips and thighs, all prime stretch-mark areas, can also help minimise the risk factors. Skin that is kept soft and supple by daily massage with a rich body cream or oil after bathing or showering is less likely to loose its elasticity than skin which is dry. Exercising during and, most important, after pregnancy will also help to keep the muscles strong and the body contours in shape, providing a taut, toned, underlying support system for the tissues as they expand and then later contract. Provided a woman is in good health, has no complications during pregnancy and receives the blessing of her doctor, she can undertake most of her normal exercise or keep-fit programme throughout almost the entire trimester. Although pregnant women can develop stretch marks at any age, there is a greater tendency for them to form either in the very young, especially during the teens, and over the age of thirty-five or forty, when skin tissue is beginning to thin and lose its natural elasticity.

Considerable evidence has come to light regarding the importance of certain vitamins and minerals in the diet in maintaining strong healthy connective tissue, which may explain why some women — possibly those who are deficient in these nutrients — are more susceptible to developing stretch marks during pregnancy than those lucky few whose bodies remain unmarred even after two or three pregnancies.

Research led by Dr Carl Pfeiffer, Director of the Brain Bio Centre in Princeton, New Jersey, indicates that human skin holds about 20 per cent of all the body's zinc, a mineral found in yeast, liver, cheese, and oysters which, with copper, to a lesser degree is needed for effective cross-linking of the elastin strands which make up perfect, firm, elastic tissue. Dr Pfeiffer believes that if these chains are imperfectly formed, overstretching, as for instance during pregnancy, will cause long tears or striae that appear as surface stretch marks. In addition to zinc, strong, prime grade elastin depends for correct synthesis on vitamin B6 — prime sources fish, meat, wheatgerm, yeast, skimmed milk and cabbage — as well as vitamin C — found in high quantities in citrus fruits and various green leafy vegetables, cabbage, and potatoes — to prevent the damaging effects of oxidation on the various enzymes involved in elastin synthesis. An increasing number of nutritionists therefore stress the importance of increasing the zinc, B6 and C in the diet during pregnancy.

. . . . . and After

The post-partum period or puerperium following childbirth is a time when the massive and sudden drop in elevated hormone levels, compounded by the stress and tiredness associated with the birth itself and the responsibility for caring for a new born infant, can take their tole on a woman's looks and well-being generally. As oestrogen and progesterone levels plummet, skin and scalp problems may flare up, temporarily, sometimes triggered by a step-up in androgen production, but these tend invariably to settle down once a woman's normal hormonal rhythms are re-established by a mechanism which at first may prove somewhat erratic, considering the disruptive impact of postnatal stress on the pituitary 'master gland' responsible for controlling and synchronising hormonal output. Very dramatic excessive hair loss is a particularly distressing postnatal disorder, a phenomenon trichologists refer to as 'post-partum *alopaecia*'. This can occur anything from two to seven months following delivery and may be so severe that many women not surprisingly are convinced they are going bald! Postnatal hair loss is, however, extremely common due to the sharp decline in oestrogen and also — sometimes rather less well known — to the fact that during pregnancy the degree of normal hair loss, amounting to an average of seventy-five hairs lost each day, is temporarily arrested or slowed down because of hormone changes, accounting for the sheen, full volume and generally improved condition of many women's hair during pregnancy. Postnatal alopaecia represents therefore a catching up on nine months of delayed normal hair loss — a quantum leap that is bound to come as a shock until you remember that new hairs are contantly replacing the old ones as they fall out. The scalp and skin generally become either very greasy or extremely dry and flaky; dandruff may break out, spots, blackheads, dingy-looking skin as well as a temporary increase or coarsening of existing facial hair add up to what certain 'new mums' during the postnatal months regard as a distinctly ugly duckling period, when many see themselves as disproportionately unattractive, their self-image distorted beyond the norm through the narrow angle lens of postnatal depression, anxiety, tiredness, irritability and over-work.

Massaging, kneading the scalp tissues to reduce muscular tension and increase the flow of blood to the tissues and hair follicles, and shampooing regularly with a mild, creamy, oil-based shampoo can greatly control scalp disorders and dandruff and regulate hair loss. Often, opting for a change in hair style, especially if this involves a switch from a long or elaborate hair style to a very short, easy-to-maintain style or cut, can work wonders in improving a woman's looks and self-confidence while encouraging faster and more profuse regrowth. A complexion that is very dehydrated should be cleansed with only the mildest and blandest of products, while a rich emollient treatment cream used night and day will counteract flakiness, prevent the formation of fine lines, and relieve tautness. Spots and blackheads should be treated with a mild antibacteria facial wash and an over-the-counter drying agent such as Topex or Oxy 5 or 10 to control grease and clogging up pores. Pregnancy or indeed the first eighteen months thereafter are most definitely not the time when any internal drugs or very potent topical ointments can be prescribed for acne, as these can have a deleterious effect on a woman's changing metabolism and, if she is breast feeding, any drugs taken during that period can, as in pregnancy, affect the immediate and future well-being of her child.

Slack, dimpled body skin, crêpiness or cellulite on thighs and buttocks can only be improved by a combination of a healthy balanced diet and a regular exercise programme to tone the muscles and help burn up the extra layers of fat laid down during pregnancy. It is worth remembering too that breast feeding doesn't benefit the baby's health exclusively but has definite advantages for the mother's rate of recovery of her former shape. Breast feeding stimulates the body to produce a powerful hormone called oxytocin — the chemical that triggers uterine contractions during birth — and gynaecologists believe this helps even after delivery to tone up the inner pelvic organs and restore normal metabolism.

It is unfortunate that the one time when a woman's figure and skin, not to mention her nerves, could greatly benefit from body massage and other beauty treatments designed to tone, tighten and refine face and body tissues as well as relax and pamper her generally is, by definition, a phase when the amount of time needed to go to a beauty salon is prohibitive and any opportunity she may have to indulge in the luxury of taking sybaritic time off is minimal. The premium of time, cost and commitment notwithstanding, the dividends paid in terms of improving body skin, body tone, greater well-being, lower stress levels, and greater self-confidence justify any amount of time invested, begged, borrowed or stolen in the first year after childbirth to invest in exercise and enjoy the occasional facial and body massage. With a newborn baby the natural and joyous centre of attention and the prime object of responsibility, the question nevertheless remains, who mothers the mother? Women with babies and young children are notoriously prone to concentrating, rightly, all their energies on the care of their infants, focusing their interest exclusively on the family and domestic environment, especially if they do not have a career to pursue, often to the total exclusion of their own needs and desires. Yet denying herself regular periods when she can rest, pamper herself, indulge in privacy, and care for her skin, body, hair, and general appearance may inevitably sow the seeds of future discontent, depression, domestic discord and rock bottom morale.

The bodily metamorphosis that occurs with pregnancy is the most dramatic one experienced in any woman's lifetime, gross illness apart. But there is no reason why, especially if she has taken care not to gain a very great amount of surplus weight or become unfit during pregnancy, a woman should not eventually with perseverance, a certain amount of discipline, and good sense regain her firmer figure after her child is born. One inspiring example of this physical metamorphosis-in-reverse can be observed in ballet dancers who possess the most steely-strong, finely tuned and yet vulnerable bodies of all and who, by staying physically active until the final stage of pregnancy and then beginning exercising again soon after delivery, build up their former strength and flexibility, reshaping their body contours down to their former spare and linear tautness.

Of all parts of the body the breasts are liable to show permanent signs of change as a result of pregnancy. The enlargement of the breasts during pregnancy is due primarily to hormonal changes, though diet can certainly help to augment the amount of fat laid down at the time. If the breasts are already large and heavy, then any extra weight will pull them down even further, so that the tissue attaching the breast to the chest wall, and the skin over the upper part of the breast, becomes stretched, causing them to sag even more. Unless the breasts are well supported at all times during pregnancy, and this goes even for women with very small breasts which can also increase greatly in volume, then distension and scarring of the skin, and drooping and sagging contours are an inevitable result. Gimmicky exercise equipment, serums, creams, massage techniques, and electronic machinery promoted as a means of reducing, lifting or tightening slack outsize breasts are often seen as a last ray of hope by many women who have lost their youthful contour, but the bottom line is that these are a complete waste of money and cannot improve the situation one iota. Since the breasts are composed entirely of fatty and glandular tissue, once this mass starts to sag, through force of gravity, and the skin becomes distended, no amount of massage or skin treatments will reverse the downward trend. Skilful cosmetic surgery to remove excess breast tissue and tighten the overlying flesh — a tricky operation at best — is about the only way to cantilever and improve the 'tilt' of the bosoms and reduce breast contours. Again, preventive measures from a very early age and especially during a first pregnancy can work wonders to minimise the deterioration of the breast shape, and this includes avoiding undue weight gain, always wearing a well-fitting supporting bra, especially while exercising, and exercising regularly to strengthen the pectoral and other muscles surrounding the breasts to counteract any tendency to droop or sag. It is also worth remembering that such commonsense measures will largely determine the upper body contours a woman is stuck with in later years.

CHAPTER 5

In Transition

Few of us relish the prospect of getting older. Throughout the centuries the mark of time has always posed different threats and fears, signifying diverse changes in the lives of each individual human being. Likewise, the chimerical quest for eternal youth goes back to time immemorial. King David slept with young virgins in the hope of absorbing their revitalising vibrations; Achilles ate the marrow of young bears to fortify his strength, while the Indian physician Susruta in 800 BC prescribed the blood and ground testicles of tigers to perk up ageing and impotent patients. Today, especially in America and increasingly in other western industrialised countries, attempts to defy old age seem to rise in direct proportion to our tendency to deify youth, and have reached obsessive proportions, which perhaps is not surprising considering that we live more than ever in an age that venerates youth, success and physical perfection — seemingly all mutually symbiotic — and old age has joined loneliness and death as modern society's last scourge and taboo.

Few would take issue with the saying that you are as old as you feel. Fair enough. But more to the point — since how we feel about ourselves greatly colours our behaviour in general — are you as old as you look? Skin, as every woman knows, is usually the first area to crack beneath the onslaught of time and, treated with scant regard, it may eventually overtake you by more than a few extra years. But dermatologists agree that a woman's skin need not and indeed does not automatically record her true chronological age — something which may work either in her favour or against it. But since skin contour and condition is something we can hardly fail to notice many times in the course of even one day, each time we glance in a mirror or when we meet other people, any degenerative changes tend to offer by far the earliest testimony of the ageing process. And so, although the spectre of old age and senility still seem light years away, the chimera of perennial youth is ultimately destined to fade away increasingly into wishful imagination.

The rate at which the skin deteriorates is certainly determined largely by heredity — dermatologists often say that in order to have youthful-looking skin for as long as possible into the forties, fifties, sixties and even seventies, you should choose your parents well. However, some of the changes in the skin such as dryness, wrinkling, cracking and chapping are truly age-related. For example, both the epidermis and the dermis become thinner as you get older, sometimes almost to the point of transparency so that the underlying veins become extremely visible. This is mainly due to the fact that skin function — just like that of every other organ in the body — inevitably slows down and becomes less efficient with age, most noticeably from the mid-fifties or early sixties onwards. Elastin synthesis ceases altogether; collagen synthesis slows down significantly, and less amount of the springy solluble collagen responsible for maintaining youthful skin is produced; skin cells are shed and renewed from the basal layers far more slowly than in youth; the moisture content of the connective tissues and epidermis diminishes steadily. The skin on the face, neck and hands, especially in people who have spent a significant amount of time out of doors and in the sun, can become blotchy, yellowy and covered in brown patches; the number of melanocytes decreases by 10–15 per cent per decade of a person's life, and it is thought that this decrease is responsible not only for the changes in hair colour as seen in elderly people but also the development of hyper or irregular pigmentation of the skin. The sebaceous glands which produce the oil that is responsible for acne also tend to diminish in number and size and greatly deccelerate their activity. The net result of this is that skin gets very much drier in older people and may become very susceptible to the effects of soap and water as well as weathering; in extreme cases, little cracks rather like crazy paving may appear on the skin which is liable to get inflamed. This very often appears on the front of the legs where the skin is very thin, especially in the winter when a person is exposed to extremes of very hot and very cold dry air. The so-called appendages of the skin also tend to diminish in number and activity with age; for instance, the sweat glands, both the eccrine variety which produce the normal watery sweat that appears on the hands and the rest of the body and also the apocrine glands, which are responsible for perspiration in the arms and the groin region, both shrink and cease to function as effectively with advancing age. The hair tends to diminish as well all over the scalp and all over the rest of the body — it is very common to find that women of sixty and more have less hair on their head and certainly far less on the body than, say, young women in their twenties. Under arms and the pubic area may become virtually denuded in men and women over the age of sixty-five or seventy. However, dermatologists and endocrinologists believe that the reduction in body and scalp hair and sometimes the increase in facial hair that is often a very distressing problem for many women as they get older may be directly related to a cut-back in hormone production — both oestrogen and the male hormone testosterone — a problem that varies very much from individual to individual and seems to be genetically predetermined and dependent largely on natural health as well as on the smooth functioning of the pituitary and the adrenal glands.

A Pause in Time

Just how gracefully any woman can hope to weather that major mid-life transition — the menopause — is something largely dictated by the whims of individual genetics, and the changes, if any, in skin appearance that occur at this time often portend just how youthful a woman can hope to remain during her fifties and even her sixties. The menopause can be described as a relatively modern condition, a time that virtually all women can expect to live through — and far beyond. But until the latter end of the nineteenth century a woman's chance of living past the age of forty-five were only 50/50. Many women died in childbirth while still fertile and others experienced a relatively short middle age. Yet modern medicine and improved nutrition has given us an average life expectancy of seventy to eighty years or more, which means that many of us can now hope to live about a third of our lives after our reproductive lifespan has ended.

But as one eminent gynaecologist puts it, nature can often be a bitch — and never more so than when controlling a woman's fundamental biology. Often euphemistically termed 'the change of life', the menopause can either signify a brief moment in time, a date on the calendar when menstruation—and fertility—come to an abrupt halt, or else an indefinitely protracted and amorphous period lasting anything from two to five years or more, accompanied by varying degrees of trauma which include hot flushes, night sweats, vaginal dryness, extreme dryness of facial and body skin, depression, irritability, and insomnia. Certainly about 50 to 60 per cent of women sail blithely through the menopause with barely a symptom of physical or emotional malaise. For the other 40 per cent or more, however, the climacteric — the term doctors use for that phase in a woman's live when her periods first become irregular or scanty until they cease altogether — can be subject to an endless barrage of physical and psychological miseries. Since the climacteric occurs most commonly between the ages of forty-five and fifty-five — sometimes earlier or a little later — it often coincides with an especially vulnerable and changeable time in life generally. Luckily, unlike some of the larger hormonal enigmas such as premenstrual tension and infertility, little mystery surrounds the menopause. Quite simply, what happens is that around the late forties or early to mid-fifties, the ovaries which have stored, ripened and released an egg each month ready for fertilisation, literally decide to shut up shop and go out of production.

During the fertile years the ovary, under instruction from the pituitary gland in the brain, produces not only the monthly egg but also the cycle of fluctuating female hormones, notably oestrogen and progesterone. With the onset of the menopause, this cycle slows down as the ovaries become increasingly resistant to messages from the pituitary gland and therefore secrete steady diminishing levels of hormones — oestrogen in particular. Oestrogen, of course, is the hormone which at puberty is responsible for giving us our femininity in the first place and for keeping the skin smooth, moist and resilient, the breasts firm and full, and lubricating the vagina, especially during sexual arousal and intercourse, during the reproductive years.

The reason why some lucky women don't suffer from sweats, flushes, dizziness, and vaginal discomfort is due to increased oestrogen output from the adrenal glands which stage a neatly balanced takeover bid that continues well into old age. It is also likely that some women's bodies adapt more smoothly and quickly to the new quota of hormones within the system. On the other hand, there is little doubt today that the most distressing and familiar menopausal symptoms are due to a severe oestrogen deficiency. In young women who have undergone a total hysterectomy — removal of both womb and ovaries — the resulting sudden oestrogen deprivation invariably results in identical but often far more acute and distressing side-effects.

The age at which a woman can expect to begin the menopause varies greatly — the widest range is between thirty-six and fifty-eight — and technically the climacteric begins with hormonal hiccups; periods either start to veer away from their established pattern, and are missed altogether, or else the time between them gets longer. It's important to remember that amenorroea — a missed period — can occur at *any* age for a variety of reasons such as a sudden emotional shock, illness, taking or coming off the Pill, prolonged stress, extreme weight loss, and of course pregnancy.

HRT — Redressing the Balance

Though British women in particular, compared to their American counterparts, may often be unaware of it, there is a very effective treatment widely available for women suffering the menopausal syndrome. Unfortunately there are still many menopausal women who, like migraine victims, tend to suffer in silent or timid ignorance of current medical developments which could ease or cure their problems.

Although there's little to commend a stoical grin-and-bear-it approach nowadays, countless women still allow themselves to be fobbed off by puritanical or ultra-conservative GPs who mete out either homespun homilies ('just your age, dear, it'll pass in time') or tranquillisers, leaving the sufferer feeling isolated, paranoid and desperate for help. Yet Valium, cups of tea and sympathetic platitudes will do little for you if you have a genuine oestrogen deficiency, and taking depressants or anti-depressants for these symptoms can damage your emotional and physical well-being without getting anywhere near the true root of the problem.

Hormone Replacement Therapy (HRT) is today the most widely recognised form of treatment for those symptoms related to oestrogen deficiency. If correctly prescribed, the side-effects are virtually non-existent. The most usual form of therapy consists of monthly courses of tablets, often in a Pill-type pack containing both oestrogen and progestogen pills, or else the insertion of a six-monthly implant beneath the skin's surface on the abdomen which gradually releases the hormones into the body.

In women whose sex drive is substantially lowered at this time, very small amounts of the male sex hormone testosterone may be prescribed also to improve libido. Oestrogen creams, jellies and pessaries are sometimes used as a back-up treatment to counteract vaginal dryness and discomfort. A simple cervical smear test will show whether a woman is oestrogen deficent (by no means all menopausal women are), and your GP should refer you to a gynaecologist or special hospital clinic who will carry this out as a routine procedure if you are between forty and fifty-five and suffering from any of the classic menopause symptoms.

While for over thirty-five years HRT has been standard treatment in America for the menopause, it is only within the past few years that this therapy has become largely accepted by the British medical profession. There is a very high success rate in preventing as well as reversing these symptoms with HRT, since physical discomfort appears to be a direct result of over-compensation by the pituitary gland for slackening oestrogen production. The basic principle of HRT is simply to boost levels of the hormone until symptoms cease, and it is regarded by British doctors ideally as short-term relief to tide over women who are going through the transitional phase.

What HRT emphatically does *not* do is act as a 'youth elixir', neither maintaining fertility nor staving off inevitable and natural signs of ageing. Nevertheless, exactly how long therapy should continue underlines the fundamental argument behind HRT. Should it be palliative or prophylactic — used preventively over possibly ten, fifteen or twenty years if a woman feels healthier and happier on oestrogen supplements? Paradoxically, while most doctors today feel morally bound to put a woman on HRT after a complete hysterectomy, few seem to regard the so-called 'natural' effects of the menopause as a suitable case for long-term treatment. Purists and 'therapy nihilists' of the old style conservative medical school still seem to regard attempts to mitigate alleged 'ageing symptoms' as fundamentally unwise, tinkering with nature, and merely delaying the inevitable. To be fair, they are also worried about the possible side-effects of long-term HRT, so exactly how safe is extended therapy?

Opponents cite the dangers of overstimulating the endometrium — the lining of the womb — with oestrogen and thus creating a threat of cancer, yet nowadays most gynaecologists are agreed that the safest form of HRT includes taking progestogen tablets in the second half of the HRT cycle to encourage a mini 'withdrawal bleed' as the womb sheds its lining, thus helping to discourage the formation of tumours. Some doctors demur, claiming that withdrawal bleeding doesn't automatically preclude irregular cell activity which could initiate benign or even malignant tumours. Others feel that few women in their fifties and sixties want the inconvenience of a monthly 'period' when all's said and done, no matter how scant.

The most convincing argument in favour of HRT in fact comes from quite a different medical camp. One of the accepted signs of ageing, particularly in post-menopausal women, is osteoporosis — weak, brittle bones caused by poor calcium absorption, which doctors have found frequently and commonly to be linked to oestrogen deficiency. Many orthopaedic specialists today therefore advocate HRT as a valuable investment policy against arm and wrist fractures, back pain, and a stooped curved spine or 'dowager's hump' — in short, to retard the annual 1 per cent rate of bone loss suffered by woman from the menopause on.

Like the tissues of the vulva and vagina, the condition of the skin, which can begin to show very definite signs of dehydration, wrinkles and dullness when oestrogen levels plummet, usually responds remarkably well to HRT, and this could well prove a crucial decision-making factor for any woman over fifty or thereabouts who is seriously alarmed at degenerative changes taking place in her skin and considering the pros and cons of HRT. What is more, a lot more than the future of her looks may be at stake. Some very recent and exciting new studies are under way at Glasgow Royal Infirmary and King's College Hospital in London which suggest that HRT not only slows down bone resorbtion and halts the rate of osteoporosis, but can prevent degenerative changes from taking place in the collagen structures of the skin. Claims that women on HRT look younger, and their skin firmer, more supple and less lined than those whose waning hormone levels are not replaced, have until now been purely anecdotal — women look more attractive, many doctors maintain, because they feel well and free from menopausal distress. But a new X-ray technique recently developed at King's College Hospital has made it possible to measure the skin's collagen content as it changes, and comparative studies show that women with low or dwindling oestrogen levels — anorexics, certain athletes, and young women suffering from amenorroea as well as menopausal women and those who have undergone a hysterectomy — suffer a progressive deterioration of collagen fibre with a particularly sharp decline in bulk two years after their last period.

That collagen synthesis should diminish along with oestrogen output makes sound sense according to John Stud, Senior Consultant in Obstetrics and Gynaecology, who, with Dr Mark Brinkat, heads the research team at King's. Fibroblasts, the master cells that manufacture collagen, have in-built oestrogen receptors that take up oestrogen as part of their normal activity, and after the ovaries cease production during the menopause, fat tissue becomes their main source of oestrogen, carrying a premenopausal 'reservoir' whose capacity is largely determined by the amount of fat cells in the body. This helps perhaps partly to explain why plumper women generally have skin that is firmer and less wrinkled than that of slimmer ones. What's more, age is irrelevant when the skin ages due to oestrogen deprivation; the skin of a forty-year-old woman experiencing a premature menopause can resemble that of a seventy-year-old if the hormonal deficit is not supplemented via another source.

Skin X-rays of women receiving HRT show that the tissues become significantly thicker after even a very short period of treatment, due to increased collagen synthesis. Under the microscope, cells taken from the vagina of older women on HRT resemble those of a young woman in the prime of her fertile years. Predictably, the King's College team, though heartened by the unexpected aesthetic bonus of HRT, are even more enthusiastic about the implication of this 'collagen link' on osteoporosis. John Studd believes that the studies contribute a giant missing piece in the puzzle of osteoporosis and why women's bones, compared to men's, should become so porous and brittle in later years. Osteoporosis, he claims, is very largely a by-product of dwindling collagen synthesis, which is the fundamental support, the latticework 'matrix' and ground substance of the body's joints and all its bony structures; decreased calcium absorption is therefore probably not, as was previously believed, the sole reason for the problem. To do your tissues — and bones — any good, HRT must be prescribed by a doctor as an internal therapy. Hormone tablets reconstitute skin from the inside out, it doesn't work the other way around, and while applying oestrogen creams around the vulva may do great things for your sex life by lubricating the inner membranes these have little cosmetic value used facially!

Diminishing Returns

No matter how fit, good looking and healthy we are, or like to *think* we are, the day-to-day reminders of age creep up on us imperceptibly, often catching us unawares, so insidious and subtly pervasive are their causes and effects. This is mainly because different parts of us age at various rates and stages, and skin ageing, far from being an isolated phenomenon, fits neatly into the overall perspective and scenario of bodily decline. When it comes down to the cellular and molecular nitty gritty, scientists have discovered that it is often the identical process of usage and abusage, environmental corrosion, and invasive inner pollution plus general wear and tear that cause stiffening and inflammation of the joints, hardening of the arteries, and loss of memory, which also account for the dehydrated, coarsened, sagging, lined and discoloured skin of men and women, in their later years.

Just why the human body, skin included, cracks up when it does, following — given a decade or so's grace, a few symptoms more or less, depending on the individual — a fairly predictable pattern, has puzzled scientists since the days of Hippocrates and Paracelsus, and undoubtedly the search for eternal or at least vastly extended youth will continue to tease and challenge man for decades to come. Nevertheless, the degeneration of skin loses much of its mystery when examined in the light of some of the current studies and recent discoveries about biological ageing.

Nowadays ageing 'theories' abound, some less plausible, well substantiated and more specious than others. 'Anti-ageing therapies' or 'life-extension systems' are an inevitable corollary, some eminently sensible in theory at any rate, others downright fanciful and way-out. What seems logical at present is that degenerative or ageing diseases are probably due to a multiplicity of interrelated factors and cannot be attributed to any one single cause. Despite the fact that gerentology (the study of the causes and effects of ageing and how to treat them) is traditionally the underfunded Cinderella of modern medicine, there is a handful of dedicated, highly respected researchers in the field today, intent on extrapolating, from the myriad factors that make our bodies tick, which ones precipitate and contribute to its demise. Most research to date has, needless to say, been carried out on laboratory animals, but allowing for the differences between mice and men there is considerable evidence that certain counter-ageing tactics — healthy diet, sufficient exercise, taking certain nutritional supplements, amending one's lifestyle — may protect homeostasis or ecological equilibrium of the body and thus militate against some of these more severe, often premature changes.

Healthy living notwithstanding, nature it seems has it in for us in a number of ways, though exactly what does us in, in the end, varies greatly from person to person. Many of today's leading scientists believe that from the moment we are born each organ of the body is programmed to slow down and eventually cease functioning at a certain pre-ordained time in our lives, a self-destruct mechanism that's genetically determined, part of an overall masterplan like what colour eyes or hair we have, and is therefore, until a miracle of genetic engineering comes along, irreversible.

Some researchers, notably Dr Leonard Hayflick Senior, Research Biologist at Children's Hospital Medical Centre in Oakland, California, believe that this clock is built into the DNA of individual cells, allowing them to divide a finite number of times after which they die. On the other hand, Dr W. Donner Denckla of the La Roche Institute of Molecular Biology, by removing the pituitary glands of laboratory animals, concludes that there is just one ageing clock centrally located in the pituitary which times the slowing down of all other parts of the body. Dr Denckla has isolated a chemical secreted by the pituitary, a sort of ageing or 'death hormone' — he calls it DECO, an acronym for 'decreasing consumption of oxygen' — which directly contributes to the degeneration of cells by interfering with the body's metabolism. The search is on to discover a DECO antibody or, better still, a blocking agent to neutralise the action of this death hormone, a breakthrough which proponents of the central ageing clock theory believe could arrest or retard many common symptoms of old age. Other scientists believe ageing — and death — are simply a natural result of wear and tear which progressively weaken the body's immunological defence system — at its peak in adolescence and in gradual decline from then on — allowing organs to become more vulnerable to attack from foreign cells, antigens and auto-immune disease, and cancer. Damage to the DNA of the cell is the basic premise underlying the 'accumulated error theory', which is based on the hypothesis that illness and pollution eventually alter the cells' genetic blueprint or 'master-plan', determining its strength and reproductive ability and overall function. DNA damage allows cells to emit false or garbled messages to one another so that they eventually become mutated, weak, and deformed, and unable to regenerate and rebuild healthy, structurally sound, tissues.

The idea that ageing results from a 'blurring' of genetic information which prevents the synthesis of top quality healthy tissues ties in rather neatly with the proposition formulating originally as far back as the 1940s by Johan Bjorksten, founder of the Bjorksten Research Foundation in Madison, Wisconsin, that defective body protein, characteristic of advancing age, is caused by the formation of cross-linking bonds or 'bridges' between protein molecules as well as between strands of RNA or DNA, which then synthesise defective proteins. Bjorksten's is the first modern theory of ageing — originally formulated because he noticed a similarity between the deterioration of duplicating film and the ageing of human skin and worked out the molecular changes responsible in both. What is more, over at the University of Nebraska School of Medicine, gerentologist Dr Denham Harman seems to have pinned down the principal culprit responsible for this cross-linkage of protein — a set of chemicals he calls 'free radicals'. Making up just two closely interlocking pieces in the very large, complex, and considerably incomplete jigsaw puzzle of ageing, the free radicals cross-linkage thesis, because it is so clearly manifested in protein, is one that casts considerable light on the nature of skin ageing in particular. For free radicals show little discrimination in their choice of targets. Faded celluloid, tanned leather, yellowed paper, rancid butter, perished rubber, rusty iron, decayed plastic, along with wrinkles, lines and crêpey skin, all testify to the all-pervasive and subversive effects of time and its triumph over organic matter. Even if it doesn't fully explain *why* skin ages when it does, the cross-linkage free radical theory all too clearly illustrates *how* it ages, because collagen comprises 40 per cent of total body protein and constitutes 80 per cent of the dermis, therefore when cross-linkage denatures its structure and cripples its synthesis, the signs of age become increasingly all too evident.

Bonds and Bridges

In youth, the collagen structures that support the skin represent a marvel of architectural symmetry. Each individual collagen strand represents a tube-like structure manufactured from a chain of amino acids, twisted into a threefold spiral-shape configuration (a triple helix), each spiral representing a unit of collagen. Numerous such units lie in neat parallel threads, and in turn these threads are laid side by side to form larger 'bundles' bound together by another protein fibre called reticulin which is partly responsible for distributing tension throughout the dermis. If you imagine a sheaf of slender asparagus stalks tightly bound up with fine strings, you will get some idea of how healthy young collagen is laid down within the connective tissues. The youth and elasticity of collagen is determined by how few bonds or cross-links as they are called attach these fibres to one another, allowing them to slide past each other with minimum restriction. Mobility and flexibility is all important, not only to the surface suppleness and smoothness of the skin but because it allows moisture, oxygen and other nutrients to travel through its network to reach the skin's cells and facilitate the excretion of waste products through the pores of the skin.

Collagen plays a tremendously important role in conserving water within the tissues. It has two types of water bonds: one variety consists of 21 per cent firmly 'bound' water and the other, more important, variety of bond contains 79 per cent free or 'swelling' water. Collagen like the rest of the connective tissues sits in a ground substance, a sort of jelly-like mixture of amino acids — mainly hyaluronic acid and mucopolysaccharides, sulphuric acid — all with tremendous water-binding powers. Two types of elastin — the other protein which is mainly responsible for keeping skin smooth and wrinkle free — short tropo-elastin and longer elastin fibres surround the collagen bundles, also weaving in and out of its network; elastin like collagen is made up of the amino acid hydroxyproline as well as arginine, lysine, glutamic acid, aspartic acid, and valine, as well as two lysine-derived amino acids, desmosin and isodesmosin. These elastin fibres, which for instance readily absorb UV-A light, are just as susceptible as collagen to the hazards of cross-linkage. Lysyl oxidase is an enzyme believed to be responsible for altering the side chains of elastin and collagen molecules causing spontaneous formulation of the cross-links which weld the fibres tighter together.

Actually, a certain amount of cross-linkage of the body's fibres is normal and necessary in order to give these protein structures their molecular order and keep the tissues in firm shape, preventing them from injury. Reticulin, which envelopes collagen fibres in a basket-like network, does so through a certain amount of cross-linkage, thereby holding the collagen bundles neatly together and giving them their shape and tension, necessary for smooth skin contours. Very soft, pliable, jelly-like foetal 'type 3' collagen, which makes up the connective tissues of babies and young children, accounts for the extreme softness and vulnerability of their skin. This is progressively replaced by adult 'type 1' collagen, tougher, firmer, but alas more susceptible to cross-linkage. In youth, however, the body produces enzymes which automatically and swiftly dismantle any superfluous cross-links. It seems that with age the ability of the body to ward off excessive cross-linking diminishes, while the rate and degree of chemical changes that accelerate cross-linkage increases. Cross-linkage within the DNA of fibroblast cells, responsible for collagen synthesis, is thought responsible for the synthesis of 'inferior' thick, non-springy protein — an increase of the amount of cross-linked 'beta chains' compared to the more youthful soluble 'alpha chains' without cross-links. As more and more cross-links form over the years, the proteinous structure underlying the skin as well as the collagen supporting the tissues of the arteries and tendons, and cushioning the joints and the bones, becomes increasingly prone to this stiffening up process. The collagen bundles become tough, less flexible and springy, losing their capacity to retain moisture — rather like old rubber. Elastin fibres, their flexibility also impaired through cross-linked bonds, become brittle, slack and over-stretched, and even snap, unable to contribute to the skin's suppleness and smoothness. Studies show that the elastin of old skin has a combination of amino acids that is significantly different from that in young people. The condition of elastin is generally regarded as a true index of skin age. For as its infrastructure degenerates, so the skin's surface reflects these changes: deepening lines, wrinkles, creases, sagging contours, and crêpiness are visible evidence that the once smooth symmetrical architecture of the dermis has begun to crumble. In the elderly, the collagen fibres tighten and shrink so much that the tiny capillaries become constricted, and the supply of blood carrying vital oxygen, moisture and nutrients is gradually cut off. The result? Inside, a tangle of disorderly, thick and hardened criss-cross protein, an internal 'frozen' metabolic pond which in turn is reflected on the outside by surface coarsening and a cross-hatch etching of lines and wrinkles.

The extent of cross-linking in skin can be measured by a simple 'pinch test' to assess the skin's mechanical properties of elasticity. Place one hand palm down on a flat surface, fingers outstretched, and grip a pinch of skin from the back of the hand with the other thumb and index finger. Hold the pinched skin for a few seconds and then release. In a young person or one who has relatively little cross-linkage of the tissues the skin will snap back instantly. In a very old person, or one whose skin has undergone premature degenerative changes, it tends to subside rather than snap back and may even show a faint ridge a few minutes later.

Under Attack

The chemical 'nasties' responsible for this foul-up are a group of high reactive substances called 'free radicals', often formed as a necessary by-product of the body's normal metabolic processes, and in the normal run of events this activity is kept in check by special neutralising enzymes, in particular sodium oxide dismutase, catalase, and peroxidase, whose job it is to deactivate these chemicals and render them harmless. But again, with age, or alternatively as the result of an extremely unhealthy lifestyle and physical neglect, the output of these protective enzymes can become sluggish, allowing these chemicals and other toxic waste to accumulate and wreak havoc in the tissues, slowing down tissue repair, or allowing only partial regeneration, attacking and damaging the fibroblast cells including eventually their DNA, thereby altering the quality of protein synthesis, and causing degenerative changes that range from wrinkles and blotchy pigmentation on the skin to more deep-seated life-threatening changes such as arteriosclerosis (hardening of the arteries) and even cancer.

But just what makes free radicals such a menace to the organism? A molecule or portion of a molecule that has become detached during a chemical reaction, a free radical usually carries one or more unpaired electrons, making it unstable, highly volatile and 'promiscuous' as it careers around the body attempting to latch onto any other molecule it can find, attacking and destroying it, and leaving mayhem and destruction in its wake. According to many a research scientist, free radicals are the principal harbingers of molecular havoc in the body.

Our bodies are constantly under siege from these noxious molecules. Sunlight in particular, cigarette smoke, alcohol, drugs, petrol fumes, ozone, and various types of radiation are just some of the recognised major sources of free radicals, as are illness, prolonged stress, and eating an unbalanced diet based largely on sweets, fats, and junk food. Because of their very high blood sugar, diabetics are more predisposed to premature collagen and elastin cross-linkage as well as to recurrent fungal yeast infections like thrush and bacterial eruptions like boils because of the skin's impaired ability to ward off infection and, scientists believe, to cope with an additional influx of free radicals. Oxygen, though the stuff of life, is in itself a prime catalyst in the release of free radicals.

One of the major sources of ageing stems from a process known as lipid peroxidation, the reaction of fats and oils with oxygen to form peroxides. A perfect example of lipid peroxidation is rancid oil or butter. The skin is the third most fatty organ of the body after the spinal chord and the brain, and it is little wonder perhaps that the effects of lipid peroxidation should manifest themselves relatively early on as wrinkles and brown 'age spots'. Known erroneously as 'liver spots' (they have absolutely nothing to do with liver function whatsoever), they are a direct by-product of lipid peroxidation and, according to some age researchers, actually represent an accumulation in skin cells (though it is thought they occur in other organs, including the brain) of a yellowish, black, granular pigment called lipofuscin which is made up largely of lipids and proteins, normal components of the cells' fatty membranes that have become oxidised, broken down by a free radical agent called malonaldehyde, and have accumulated over the years as a sort of cellular 'garbage'. Lipofuscin can eventually take up as much as 30 per cent of the cells' volume, accounting for the smattering of age pigments on the face, neck, and in particular backs of hands of men and women in their late fifties, sixties and seventies.

The cross-linkage theory of ageing with free radicals and peroxidation cast as the main villains of the piece is a particularly appealing one to many scientists, largely because there exists a formidable battery of both natural and synthetic substances noted for their purported ability to counteract the effects of oxidation. Dermatologists and scientists whose chief study is the degeneration of connective tissue, arteries, muscles, and protein fibre, see the protective role of these sundry 'antioxidants' and 'free radical deactivators' as they are called as fundamental in the battle against ageing, with the result that certain nutrients such as vitamins C,E, zinc and selenium are regarded by many nutritionists and 'holistic' health practitioners as essential for the upkeep of healthy youthful skin. To date, however, most of the claims made for the anti-ageing properties of these substances remain woolly and unsubstantiated, whatever little published data there is offering inconclusive evidence based on rather tenuous limited experiments carried out on laboratory animals only. While it makes sense, in theory at any rate, to take nutritional supplements recognised for their antioxidant and generally protective properties — provided these have been proven safe and an optimum dose is adhered to — there is no evidence whatever that when ingested, these substances actually reach the desired target site within the cell or tissues so that they can do any good. Following the principle, however, that protection and prevention is the best policy when attempting to retard the ageing process, Dr Denham Harman of the University of Nebraska School of Medicine stresses that there are three ways in which he believes we can defend ourselves against free radical damage: (a) stay thin; eat less to reduce the output of free radicals created via metabolism; (b) eat fewer polyunsaturate fats, a prime target of oxidation; (c) add free radical scavengers such as vitamins C,E, A, B6 and BI, zinc, selenium, BHT, and cysteine to the diet to mop up and neutralise any aberrant molecules.

In support of his claim, Dr Harman has demonstrated that feeding weaned mice on diets supplemented by antioxidants increased their lifespan by 30–40 per cent — 100 years in human terms. Free radical 'scavengers' or deactivators act as blocking agents, reacting harmlessly with destructive molecules before they have a chance to attack any part of the body. Antioxidants supposedly slow down the peroxidation of lipids, usually by allowing themselves to be oxidised and thus using up oxygen before it can react adversely with lipids in the system. Very often one substance such as vitamin E will be an all-in-one anti-oxidant-cum-free-radical deactivator, since one action usually potentiates the action of the other, i.e. peroxidation results in the formation of free radicals. Many natural and synthetic or man-made molecules work together synergistically (each contributing to the other one's action), as for example vitamin E and selenium, vitamin C and zinc.

Again, it cannot be stressed strongly enough that to date, such extravagant claims remain largely unsubstantiated, and reaction from the medical profession at large ranges from mild scepticism to a mighty roar of disgust and dissension that all talk of anti-ageing substances and the existence of so-called life-enhancing nutrients is sheer hokum.

Natural Antioxidants/Free Radical Deactivators

Vitamin C
A substance essential to life, like oxygen and water, this is the one vitamin that even some doctors agree can help the body ward off infection, speed wound healing, and detoxify the blood stream. C plays an integral role in collagen synthesis and also protects fatty tissues from oxidation damage. Lack of vitamin C can cause skin lesions to heal slowly, encourages anaemia (C is necessary for proper assimilation of iron), makes the skin more prone to bruising and dehydration, and leads to slack muscle tone. Taken in megadoses, nutritionists believe it can rapidly neutralise and flush out accumulated toxins in the system, and large doses of C are often prescribed routinely to accelerate detoxification in cases of alcohol poisoning. Humans, along with guinea pigs and other primates, are unique in that they do not manufacture C in the body as other animals do, and so a regular nutritional supply is vital to good health. Total deficiency or deprivation leads to scurvy, including cracked lips, bleeding gums, and skin sores.

Vitamin E
This has unfortunately attracted much sensationalistic press coverage in recent years as the 'sex vitamin', following studies

which indicate that rats deprived of vitamin E become sterile. Actually while claims that E raises libido are distinctly dubious, the protective benefits it confers against heart disease, thrombosis and strokes are more credible, due to its anti-coagulant (anti-blood clotting) properties. An important natural antioxidant, vitamin E is at present the only known antioxidant that prevents peroxidation not only of the cell membrane but also of the microsomes and mitochondria within the cytoplasm itself. It is therefore regarded by many researchers as a powerful ally of healthy cellular metabolism, reinforcing cells and tissues against attacks from free radicals and peroxidation. In Russia, experiments show that giving large doses of vitamin E and A to elderly people seems to help in reducing facial wrinkles as well as increasing energy, improving memory and concentration, and sleeplessness. The benefits of vitamin E are heightened by combining it with other antioxidants such as cysteine and selenium; nutritionists suggest a daily maintenance dose of between 400–800 international units (IU) a day.

Selenium
This is a trace element which has only recently generated much scientific interest regarding its protective role against heart disease. Toxic when taken in doses even just a few times higher than those needed for optimum health, it works best in conjunction with vitamin E and is purportedly a powerful antioxidant and free radical inhibitor. Selenium is a co-factor in the protective enzyme gluthionine peroxidase which neutralises lipid peroxides.

Enzymes
Working on the premise that the damage wrought to protein is often caused or exacerbated by dwindling enzyme production as we age, the concept of boosting enzymes makes sense in the fight against ageing. In young healthy skin, one which is not unduly bombarded with too much sunlight or pollutants, damage to the cells' DNA — which in its spiral helices contains the blueprint or working copy of all information the body's cells and tissues need to reproduce themselves and function correctly — is regularly repaired with masterly precision. This process is known as 'excision repair'; when a section of one of the twisted spirals that make up the DNA becomes damaged, special repair enzymes

secreted by the cell come to the rescue, by cutting out the damaged segment, rather like a plumber removing a broken section of pipe, and promptly re-synthesising a new section, thus preventing faulty cell reproduction.

Scientists are currently attempting to isolate and synthesise certain enzymes or else find ways to restimulate their production. Some enzymes, they believe, could even help to undo the damage of cross-linkage in the tissues. For example, a group of enzymes called elastases are known to dissolve elastin in the connective tissues, while others dissolve old collagen in the uterus after pregnancy. Beta-aminopropionitrite (BAPN), derived from the chick pea, inhibits cross-linkage in newly formed elastin and collagen, and a microbial enzyme isolated by Johan Bjorksten at the Upjohn Company, called Bacillus Cereus, has been found to work in a similar way. Decreased collagen cross-linkage is one of the side-effects in animals when they are injected with penicillamine, an amino acid derived from penicillin which is also used as a chelating (binding) agent to draw excess levels of dangerous metals out of the body. Tropical fruits such as papaya (papaw) and pineapple contain very high quantities of the proteolytic (protein digesting enzymes) papain and bromelain, which are known to digest about thirty-six times their own weight in protein. Both substances have been identified as anticross-linking agents. Some researchers believe that eaten fresh and in high quantities these fruits can help to guard against excessive tissue damage. Applied directly to the skin, they can also speed healing of wounds and blemishes by boosting the skin's natural self-repair mechanism, though it's doubtful that tropical fruit can work similarly to prevent lines and wrinkles.

An enzyme which has been the subject of much publicity recently as a possible 'youth elixir' is sodium oxide dismutase (SOD), just one of the hundreds of enzymes produced by the body to process harmful chemical waste including superoxides. Although marketed in Britain and America as a nutritional supplement to ward off the ravages of oxidation and ageing, controversy hinges on whether SOD taken internally ever gets to the site where all the action is — right inside the cell. The late Dr Benjamin Frank reported considerable success in 'rejuvenating' wrinkled, slack, hyper-pigmented skin, greying hair and other organic symptoms of ageing with intensive therapy combining SOD with foods high in nucleic acids — for example, sardines, and oily fish, raw vegetables, vegetables juices and fruit, the richest source of natural enzymes to boost the cellular cell-repair mechanism.

Amino Acids

These are the building blocks from which the body constructs its protein. Those thought to offer most protection against peroxides and free radicals are the sulphur-based amino acids, taurine, methionine, and cysteine, the most powerful of all three because it neutralises acetaldehyde, a potent toxin present in cigarette smoke, smog and alcohol. Eggs are the richest source of sulphur amino acids as well as the most perfect balance of dietary protein.

Deanol (DNAE)

Marketed in America under the trade-name Deaner, this is a precursor of the vitamin choline and, according to studies, is directly absorbed by the cell membrane, where it acts as a powerful free radical scavenger helping to break up the accumulation of the age pigment lipofuscin in the cell. Oily fish such as sardines and mackerel are the greatest source of deanol and choline. Centrophanoxine is a derivative of DNAE and has been used medically in Europe with considerable success to treat general ageing symptoms such as speech and motor dysfunction, loss of memory, and other cerebral problems linked to ageing. American experiments with laboratory animals suggest that injections of centrophanoxin can prolong their lifespan and also fade accumulation of lipofuscin in the cells by stimulating their natural ability to demolish free radicals.

Synthetic Compounds

In addition to these vitamins, minerals, enzymes and other basically natural substances acknowledged for their antioxidant properties, in recent years some American gerentologists have turned their interests towards a most unlikely alternative source of anti-ageing substances — chemical food preservatives. To a certain extent it may seem logical enough rather than incongruous that chemicals which are used to decrease the rate of oxidation in stored food may serve a similar purpose in the human body, though evidence of this is at best flimsy. Gerentologists are testing certain compounds in both animals and humans to find out whether they do have any real value in promoting longevity and preventing premature ageing symptoms, but to date all claims as to their rejuvenating powers are largely speculative. What is more, very little is known about the hidden health hazards of taking these chemicals, especially in doses large enough to have any impact on the system. Some cases of allergic sensitivity, including dermatitis in humans and liver, kidney and thyroid changes in animals, have been reported after these drugs were administered over long periods. Anti-cancer properties have been attributed to two such chemicals, BHT and BHA, both powerful peroxides and free radical inhibitors. Dr Denham Harman believes that large doses of BHT could add at least five years to the average human lifespan. Some researchers have discovered that in albino hairless mice, BHT reduces the incidence of skin cancer induced by ultraviolet light, and others have found it effective against viruses including herpes simplex. Other chemicals attracting attention as potential youth drugs include ethoxyquin, whose metabolic activity is similar to that of vitamin E and is used to prevent oxidation of sliced fruit and animal feeds: thiodlpropionic acid, used to stabilise vitamins and antibiotics and prevent flavour changes in milk products and soya bean oil; and nordihydroguaiaretic acid (NDGA), a resinous substance derived from plants including the creosote bush and guaiac gum trees, and used as an antioxidant in piecrusts, sweet lard, butter, and ice cream.

The idea that stuffing one's face with such exotic-sounding substances, which prolong the life and stabilise the condition of food, might also one day keep human tissue in tip-top prime condition — in a sense prolonging the shelf life of man — does rather strain the bounds of credibility. But then it is worth remembering that the idea of using common or garden novocaine — the very same pain killer used by dentists — to treat symptoms of ageing must have seemed just as derisory a few decades ago, when the concept was first introduced. The apparently impressive results of gerovital H.3 in treating both the physical and mental stresses of ageing were common knowledge in eastern Europe long before the therapy found popularity in the West. Gerovital H.3 was originally developed by Dr Ana Aslan, a Rumanian gerentologist, who quite by chance discovered that a combination of novocaine and a mixture of potassium benzoic salts and other trace elements and minerals had an instantaneous and often long-term effect on many degenerative ailments.

Reports indicate that GH 3 tones up the central nervous system and therefore seems particularly effective in tackling the more psychosomatic elements of ageing including depression, insomnia, anxiety, irritability, poor memory and concentration, and general sexual problems, while other therapists have for quite some time now been prescribing gerovital successfully for menopausal symptoms as well as for the more general effects of stress such as fatigue, drug addiction, illness in relatively young men and women, the premature ageing of the skin and hair and nail problems.

Although scientists are optimistic they will come up with a breakthrough in the battle against ageing within the next five years, as yet none of the antioxidants or free radical deactivators that make news from time to time carry any credibility in medical circles, since there has been minimal published documentation and research is as yet confined to the test tube or laboratory rodents, making the prospect of perennially wrinkle-free skin, firm connective tissue, flexible, well-toned muscles and arteries as elusive and unattainable a dream as it ever was. Short of committing our bodies to deep-freeze storage — a rising trend in some circles in certain parts of America — there is little chance of giving old age the slip entirely, and the most we can hope for is to die reasonably good looking and in reasonably good shape.

CHAPTER 6
The Rejuvenation Game

That skin care is no longer regarded a luxury but an everyday necessity by millions of women is reflected in very revealing consumer and market trends. Skin alone accounts for one seventh of our annual expenditure on all beauty and toiletry items and is rising steadily. British women spent 422 million pounds on skincare and make up in the year ending June 1984, 36 million pounds up on the previous year, with the result that its embellishment and so-called rejuvenation have in the past few decades spawned multi-million-dollar cosmetics industries in America, Europe and developed countries the world over. The beauty business is one of the most colourful, challenging yet ultimately confusing markets in the world today. It is obvious when you observe the sophisticated advertising, self-styled apostles, and well-orchestrated trends, that youth, like sex, sells, and the beauty industry, rubbing shoulders with show business, represents a last glamorous niche of never never land that still trades largely in illusion, ephemera, and dreams that might just come true for anyone with sufficient money and time and a disbelief-system well enough suspended to indulge in them. How could the cosmetics industry flourish as it does if hope, let alone vanity, did not spring eternal?

For as the French writer Stendhal observed, beauty is often the mere promise of happiness, a promise so powerfully seductive and beguiling that it rarely fails to elicit belief, if only subliminally, from even the most sceptical of customers. Ageless perfect skin is, after all, the implicit *sine qua non* behind each new skin-cream, lotion and bar of soap launched on an ever-susceptible market. To the majority of consumers of all ages, from fifteen to seventy-five, the world of cosmetics and beauty treatments remains a perplexing jungle. The beauty editor of any glossy woman's magazine can testify to the fact that it is ingeniously laid with mines ready to trap any hapless woman (or indeed man) unfamiliar with its exotic terrain. Thanks to media hype, and the quasi-scientific jargon coined by beauticians and manufacturers touting their newest treatments, the science of skin care has fast become blurred by half-baked facts and fallacies. The catechism of eternal youth strikes a chord as hollow yet salutary as the tale of the emperor's new clothes. So are the cosmetic manufacturers really having us on?

Giving Nature the Slip

The question of whether today's expensive, glossily packaged skin-care products have any real value whatever in retarding skin ageing and reducing lines and wrinkles, or whether indeed they are any more efficient than the cheaper, less glamorous brands at the 'bottom end' of the market, makes up a long-standing and familiar polemic argued *ad nauseam* by cosmetic manufacturers on the one hand, and doctors and chemists on the other. When we pay the exorbitantly high prices charged by the big manufacturers, are we paying mainly for the glossy packaging, the lavish ads and in-store promotions, or for exclusive special ingredients that can purportedly stave off the onslaught of time? Spokesmen for the major companies like Revlon, Lancôme, Orlane, and Estée Lauder rarely deny that the answer is both, but they stress that profits are ploughed back into extensive research into the nature of skin ageing, research which often leads cosmetic chemists to join forces with specialists working in fields as diverse as rheumatology, immunology, cardiovascular disease, nutrition etc., isolating and synthesising anti-ageing substances, and developing and testing products of the very highest quality that they claim can help to retard or reverse the causes and effects of skin ageing. But how credible are the claims, and what use if any are the creams?

Whether cosmetics can or cannot penetrate beyond the epidermal barrier and get to work on living skin cells is what the whole issue really boils down to. In recent years the question has been aired in heated debate in the press, radio, TV and in special consumer programmes bent on exposing corruption within the beauty business! Dermatologists tend to remain scathing in their response to claims that certain products and ingredients have a regenerative effect on living tissues. They argue unequivocally that since skin provides an impermeable barrier against externally applied substances, creams and lotions can only be absorbed by the uppermost layer of dead cells and as such have no access to the dermal layers where the skin cells renew themselves. The corollary to this argument is that because they cannot travel beyond the epidermis, any exotic age-retarding ingredients are automatically rendered useless, and therefore a simple product such as lanolin, petroleum jelly or baby lotion will do every bit as well to soften and protect the skin's surface.

But then the relative permeability of the skin presents a vexing question as yet unresolved even within certain circles of the medical profession. On the one hand, skin is used as a vehicle in the new trans-epidermal drug delivery systems: medication such as nitroglycerine for heart disease, which would otherwise be taken orally, is now alternatively prescribed in the form of an impregnated stick-on plaster to be released slowly into the system. On the other, the dangers of systemic absorption and the resulting suppression of the immune system inherent in the over-use of potent corticosteroid ointments have been well established, while the reason that anti-androgen creams work to clear up acne and suppress hair loss in some people is because they penetrate into the living cell structure of the pores and follicles. Clearly therefore there *is* sufficient proof that skin can, albeit selectively, absorb certain substances beyond the epidermal barrier, but whether cosmetic ingredients can be included in that select group remains largely a matter for conjecture, since proof, if indeed there is any, is hard to find. Apart from radioactive tagging of certain substances to measure penetration, and the use of dansylchloride, an invisible dye, to identify the supposedly accelerated renewal rate of skin cells, no cosmetic company has as yet been able to offer a smidgeon of conclusive scientific evidence that any ingredient can cause a meaningful change in skin cell physiology. Reports on skin improvement as a result of using new products are invariably subjective, since it is impossible to do histological (i.e. tissue culture) analysis of each woman's skin before and after the testing period. What is more, according to top dermatologists like Dr Albert Kligman of the University of Pennsylvania, even if one were to believe the spurious claims that substances can penetrate living tissue, it is unclear what they would do once they *got there*. This seems a very reasonable caveat.

It is highly doubtful whether any of the antioxidants, free radical inhibitors, proteins, amino acids, vitamins, cellular extracts etc., could ever zero in on the requisite target site within and around the actual cells themselves to strengthen their reproductive capacity, repair and combat the damage brought by UV light, oxidation, and free radicals, and improve the water-binding properties of the connective tissue. Cosmetics, after all, are not drugs. If they were, you would have to get them on prescription from your GP. Mucopolysaccharides, hyaluronic acid, elastin, collagen, are just some of the ingredients synthesised from a panoply of known skin constituents, but the rationale for their inclusion in cosmetics seems spurious, to say the least. Like every other organ, system, or tissue in the body, skin is constantly being reconstituted and repaired, new tissue synthesised, fluid replaced from *within* via the continuous metabolic processes responsible for maintaining homoeostasis or all-round physical health. No one would argue that young firm radiant and smooth skin is indeed vitally dependent on moisture, a sufficient supply of oxygen-rich blood to its surface, strong flexible capillary walls, steady cell turnover, unimpaired collagen and elastin synthesis, and the destruction of free radicals by the body's own warrior enzymes. But these functions are a fundamental part of human biology and thus unlikely to be greatly affected by the application of creams and serums spiked with exotic ingredients.

Proof — The Mighty Molecule

Prime examples are the ubiquitous collagen and elastin without which it seems no self-respecting hi-tech anti-ageing skin cream of the 1980s would be complete. Collagen and elastin, according to many a press 'blurb', are included to replenish the skin's own protein fibres, repairing damage and augmenting their structure, moisture content, suppleness and elasticity. Not so, say scientists. Both elastin and collagen are composed of peptide chains whose molecular weight is too heavy and whose dimension too big to penetrate the epidermis. The molecular weight of collagen is 300,000, yet as nothing over 70,000 can penetrate the skin, these proteins must be hydrolysed — broken down — and made soluble so that they can be incorporated into cream and emulsion which will penetrate the upper skin layer. Thus chopped up, processed and reconstituted, this 'soluble' collagen used in cosmetics bears about as much resemblance to the protein fibres which make up our connective tissue as a cube of hydrolysed beef extract does to a sirloin steak! Where soluble collagen and elastin can help to improve the quality of the skin, however, is by improving its surface softness, helping to regulate the evaporation of moisture from the epidermal cells and so preventing dehydration. In other words, elastin and collagen can improve the texture and emollient quality of skin creams. Any good moisturising cream or fluid — in essence a judicious blend of oils, waxes, fats, humectants and water, smoothly and well stabilised (i.e. emulsified) against separation, with just the right ratio of oil to water, emollient yet not too tacky and greasy — will cover the epidermis with a light occlusive barrier to prevent moisture loss and soften the dead dry surface cells and plump them out so that lines and wrinkles *appear* fewer and less clearly or deeply defined; surface coarseness, dryness and 'pull' is also instantly relieved. 'Temporary rejuvenating' effects are purely illusory. The skin can *look* younger though it isn't. And who indeed could ask for more? Once it has formed, a line is a line, a wrinkle a wrinkle, destined to stay there for good — though proper skin care, protection against sunlight, and the use of moisturisers especially in a very harsh dry environment can certainly prevent more from forming in too rapid a succession or indeed prematurely.

Great Expectations

Simone de Beauvoir once stated that we should bow to age; Anaïs Nin, another feminist writer, said that on the contrary we should transcend it. Two diametrically opposing viewpoints, both equally valid, both exemplifying the vastly different emotions inspired by the passage of time and its effects on the body. What we spend and expect from our cosmetics is determined largely by the degree of importance we attach to the formation of wrinkles and whether we regard the natural changes in skin with fear or equinimity or even pride. This in turn calls into question the accepted criteria for youthfulness and attractiveness put across by the media and advertising. The apotheosis of the twenty-five-year-old girl as the epitome of true beauty, femininity and desirability is one of the most powerful images and marketable commodities ever fabricated within the advertising industry. Largely illusory, almost totally unrealistic, it remains nevertheless today's 'ideal', calculated to tease and titillate, especially those women gripped by the paranoia of ageing and motivated through neurotic compulsive tendencies to spend hundreds upon hundreds of pounds each year on new skin products, ever hopeful, ever obsessed by the belief that out there, there may be a new miracle ingredient, product or treatment that can put back or halt the clock, or allow them to come closer to attaining this ultimate ideal of beauty. For the sad thing about this paranoid obsession with every little line, crease and wrinkle as it begins to form, the agonising searching and resulting depression or anxiety that accompanies a woman's ritual close-up consultation with her magnifying mirror is that, like the anorexic teenager who perceives a totally misconstrued, inaccurate image of her body, any woman who focuses only on her facial or epidermal defects and magnifies them out of all proportion to her overall appearance, builds up a warped self image, noticeable only to herself. In the end, how you stand on the issue of those dreaded, inevitable wrinkles depends very largely on whether *you* consider them ugly and unsexy or rather a perfectly normal representation of character, a testimony to a life well lived, experienced and enjoyed, and as such an enhancement not a negation of beauty. The number of men of all ages who find laugh lines, for example, extremely attractive and even sexy in a woman is salutary proof that sexual attractiveness, femininity and vibrant beauty are not necessarily always synonymous with a line-free, baby-smooth complexion. Even the late Elizabeth Arden was once prompted to say that a face without lines is like a book without words (possibly meant as balm for those customers who found her cosmetics did less than expected for their lines?), and a blank expression, no matter how aesthetically perfect and conventionally beautiful is a little bizarre and disconcerting on any woman past her twenties or thirties and certainly her forties, and has little to do with the true, overall beauty or attractiveness that stems from inner vitality, sexuality, strength, personal style, wisdom, and humour, as well as from a beautiful skin.

So why be afraid of wrinkles? Learning to apply make-up skilfully ensures that few people other than the individual concerned may even be aware of them. A prime example is that applying expert eye make-up to make the most of the size and the shape of the eyes can dramatically undermine the impact of fine laugh lines and crow's feet round the eyes. It is worth remembering too that most people do *not* evaluate another person's attractiveness or youthfulness by peering intently at and counting up every wrinkle, pore and crease on their face. The impact and impression we make, whether favourably or less so, on others is made up by the sum total of various parts, and the sum is inevitably *greater* than those parts. Women do not usually inspire admiration, engender popularity or become objects of male desire and love, just because of one or two isolated attributes such as long lustrous hair, long legs, slim thighs, a taut tummy, or a creamy magnolia complexion. The *overall* aspect and appearance is what gives us our image and helps others to formulate their opinion of personality, looks and age. For instance, a few crow's feet around the eyes, and nose-to-mouth laugh lines or a cross-hatch of expression lines on the forehead, are not nearly as ageing or noticeable to others as an expression of tension, fatigue, anger or discontent which pulls the face along a downward gradient, of the gauntness or droopy, loose and untoned facial and neck contours which may result from persistent dieting and extreme weight changes. A flabby untoned body, becoming noticeably overweight, acquiring poor posture, and slow or tense movements, indicative of an inactive, sedentary lifestyle, all can and do add years to a person's true age, regardless of whether they have wrinkles or not. Similarly, it is one of the laws of nature that facial and bodily contour changes — extreme weight gain, (or extreme weight loss), flabby muscles, swollen puffy tissues, bags under the eyes, a lax jaw line, jowls or a double chin, facial creases and folds — are far more ageing than any number of wrinkles if they appear on the surface of fundamentally taut, well-toned flesh. Therefore appraising lines and wrinkles as they form *in perspective* to one's overall appearance is far more likely to yield a realistic picture of the true nature of the ageing process than a neurotic obsession with fine detail that no one else would ever notice. And, when it comes to the crunch, what about those much neglected wrinkles of the mind, often more ageing than those of the face and body? In the end, age is as much a state of mind as of body.

Illusion — Cause and Effect

That cosmetics — skin-care products and make-up — can and do make women more attractive is a fact few people would dispute. Since many centuries BC women and men of ancient civilisations acknowledged the sexual, social, aesthetic and even political powers of adornment of the face, recognising that the skilled use of cosmetics provides a powerful and simple means to manipulate what we look like and so determine the messages we transmit about ourselves. But the important role that cosmetics play in health care is only now beginning to be recognised and evaluated, thanks to exciting pioneer work now underway in Britain and America to establish the psychotherapeutic value of cosmetics amongst healthy women of all ages as well as those suffering from emotional and physical problems.

Dr Jean Ann Graham has recently conducted some interesting studies that corroborate what most women have always known or instinctively believed anyway: that the more attractive you are, the higher your self-esteem. Psychological research shows that the level of a person's physical attractiveness or unattractiveness has profound and significant social implications in all areas of life. These studies suggest that the advantages enjoyed by attractive people are numerous and include greater self-esteem and confidence, and the ability to be more outgoing, to obtain better jobs and do better in interviews, to attract friends, help, and guidance, to marry into a higher social class, and to be excused for any negative feelings. The physically attractive are also more favourably rated on what is known as personality attributes including kindness, sociability, and sensitivity. Dr Graham, who obtained her Ph.D. from the Department of Experimental Psychology at Oxford and now works in close collaboration with Dr Albert Kligman at the University of Pennsylvania, Department of Dermatology, hypothesises that since cosmetics improve attractiveness, the corollary is that their use should engender enhanced self-perception, particularly important, she stresses, in promoting psychological well-being as ageing progresses and during treatment for physical and mental illness. She has conducted a number of studies to prove this point. In a series of control studies involving elderly women from their sixties to their nineties, some hospitalised, and women of all ages suffering emotional disorders, Dr Graham demonstrated that teaching women who hitherto had not used cosmetics or skin-care products to apply make-up and care for their skin made an appreciable difference to their self-esteem, sense of optimism and general attitude to life. These 'make overs' confirmed earlier findings that physically attractive and unattractive elderly females perceive themselves differently. More attractive women see themselves as healthier and have a more positive outlook on life, are more optimistic, less depressed, and better adjusted. Look good and the chances are you are also more satisfied with your lot in life and more involved and more realistic.

In control studies to assess the value of make overs (i.e. giving women a facial treatment and applying make-up as a means both of showing how cosmetics can improve their looks, while teaching them how to apply them themselves), not surprisingly perhaps those women who were relatively unattractive improved significantly more in terms of self-confidence, cheerfulness, and optimism than the more attractive, since the changes in their appearance and thus in their self-perception were more noticeable and dramatic. More heartening still in terms of long-term effects, the self-perception of the 'low physical attractiveness' groups also improved more than that of the better-looking women, while they also continued to use cosmetics at least one month after the initial make over. The results suggest that the more room there is for improving one's looks, the greater and more longlasting will be the aesthetic and psychological benefits — at any age.

Although the pioneer work of Dr Graham and Dr Kligman represents exciting exploratory research in a very new field, it is already becoming clear that psychotherapeutic cosmetology may grow into an important adjunctive therapy in the treatment of any number of physical, mental and age-related disorders. In Britain, since the 1950s, the work of the Red Cross in helping men and women overcome the physical defects resulting from burns, plastic surgery, birth deformities such as port wine stains, disfiguring skin diseases such as vitiligo, as well as chronic sickness, through teaching techniques of applying camouflage make-up and providing general grooming, hair and skin care has grown steadily. The old adage that a person will feel good if they look good is often dismissed as an empty cliché, yet it now seems to have far reaching and profound implications for the health of the elderly and the sick. But if better self-esteem, self-image and confidence, the desire to go out and socialise, contentment to look at one's self in the mirror and other optimistic attitudes towards one's self and life generally can be generated through teaching women to make the best of themselves by learning to use cosmetics, then the value of cosmetic therapeutic intervention, as Dr Graham calls it, knows no bounds, since it addresses itself to improving the quality of an ageing or sick person's life — an amorphous area, often ignored by the medical profession who are, it seems, often merely interested in prolonging life at the expense of its quality. As the Philadelphia team have confirmed, by acting as a vehicle to reach a person's subconscious, cosmetics can prove as powerful as the most potent systemic drug or medicine — and without any of the side-effects!

It follows that if a person's motivation to improve her appearance and self-image are low because of illness, then this could easily lead to a self-perpetuating negative mind/body/mind cycle, whereby low self-esteem leads to further neglect of appearance, and negative responses from other people, and so full recovery from illness is delayed or halted. Therefore, says Dr Graham, cosmetic intervention can be used *curatively* — to generate the development of a positive feedback cycle in depressed patients or those recovering from illness or surgery, who have a poor self-image — as well as in a *preventive* way to help maintain positive mental attitudes and esteem or prevent the impending onset of a negative cycle. Experiments carried out in the late 1960s on the effects of performing plastic surgery on criminals with disfigured faces, show that removing scars, tattoos etc., has a considerable affect on the recidivism rate.

As the role of cosmetics — both corrective (to minimise ageing, skin diseases and blemishes such as acne) and standard (to improve general appearance and attractiveness) is appreciated more fully, closer collaboration between cosmetic companies, dermatologists, psychologists, psychiatrists, hospital staff and beauticians, and health workers is bound to revolutionise both the world of health care and of beauty therapy, and even of cosmetics. At the moment Britain leads the field, having founded the cosmetic camouflage service in 1975, a volunteer service formed under the auspices of the British Red Cross to which doctors and surgeons can refer patients who require corrective cosmetic treatment for specific skin defects, or to aid in the treatment of psychological disorders. Instruction in the psychological principles underlying these treatments is now being incorporated into the Red Cross treatment programme. Red Cross volunteers — who have, sad to say, as yet no counterpart, for example, in America and Canada — work mainly in psychiatric maternity and geriatric wards, and in homes for the elderly, and undergo intensive training in the skills required to administer fundamental beauty treatments, such as manicures, facial skin care, massage of the neck, shoulders and hands, hair care and make-up.

CHAPTER 7
True to Type

Skin pigment is the imprint that more than any other genetic marker immediately and vividly identifies our racial origins, though the accepted definitions of skin tone and type have, in the second half of the twentieth century alone, become less clear cut, encompassing new subtleties and nuances of tone. As societies throughout the western world and industrialised countries have become heterogeneous, inter-racial marriages have resulted, often producing stunningly exotic and beautiful genetic 'permutations' as the hybrid varieties of black, brown, olive, and fair skins become ever more infinite and the subtleties of polymorphous pigmentation infinitely more interesting. Such overlap and melding is not without its own set of problems. The idiosyncracies previously endemic in one race may be inherited just as easily by another along with other aesthetic qualities. The simplest method of defining these various indigenous quirks and qualities is, however, still to divide the skin into its most easily recognisable types.

Fair/Celtic Skin

This is characteristically accompanied by red, blond or 'mousy' brunette hair and grey, green or blue eyes, and is often prone to freckles. Admired the world over for the translucence and fragile, porcelain quality of their skin, fair-skinned men and women, especially those who make up a large part of the population of hot sunny countries like South Africa, New Zealand, Australia, and parts of America, run the greatest danger of severe sunburn, premature ageing and skin cancer, because of insufficient melanin synthesis, the skin's natural defence to sunlight. People with red hair and freckles are particularly at risk, because the few melanocytes they do have are unevenly distributed and clumped together. The fair skin typically burns, with all the attendant ugliness and discomfort, and often fails to develop a tan — not such a mystery, because burning and tanning are totally separate and different mechanisms. To avoid cancer, premature ageing, wrinkles, lines, loss of elasticity, solar keratoses (non-malignant wart-like growths), brown blotches and yellow hyper-pigmentation, a classic sign of solar elastosis or severe sun damage, the best policy is to stay out of the sun or wear a sunscreen with a PF of 15 or more or a total sunblock to prevent the pain and damage caused by burning. Fair skin is usually thinner than its olive counterpart and may have less underlying cutaneous tissue and fewer and less active sebaceous glands. It is therefore prone to dehydration, irritation from effects of the weather, and the formation of natural expression lines and creases and so requires assiduous moisturising, conditioning care, and protection from the elements.

Olive/Mediterranean Skin

Characteristic of Italy, Spain, France, Greece and the countries ranging as far east as Turkey and North Africa and south as South America, the skin tones are a composite of yellow sometimes reddish pigment, very often prone to ashy sallowness when not exposed to sunlight, and with a predominant tendency to oiliness though rarely to spots, blackheads and acne. Like its darker cousin the 'Latin' complexion is fundamentally a hardy one that ages later and less noticeably than the Celtic or northern skin. Body and facial contours are often plumped out by an additional layer of fat, lubricated by sebaceous secretion, and protected from ultraviolet light damage by the ability to tan deeply and quickly without burning. Excess facial as well as profuse body hair can be a problem of this skin type, often more noticeable because growth is dark and coarser than in fairer people. Hair around the nipples, between the breasts, on the bikini line and upper lip need regular and efficient depilation such as waxing or electrolysis to maintain smoothness and weaken hair growth. However, in certain countries in the Mediterranean, as in Islamic countries, body hair in women is still regarded by both sexes as sexually attractive, even though many women omit shaving areas such as underarms at the expense of personal freshness and hygiene.

Asian/Oriental Skin

Predominantly yellow in tone or very pale with a tendency to sallowness, the Japanese, Chinese or Asian skin suffers from fewer indigenous problems than any other racial type. Physiognomy — skin stretched taut over a flattish bone structure and a limited repertoire of facial expressions, giving a relatively inanimate, inscrutible appearance — seems to defy the accepted lines, creases, folds and slackness of age as we recognise them, and it is sometimes impossible accurately to assess the age of oriental or Asian men and women. Moreover, in the east, blemishes and unaesthetic skin conditions are the exception rather than the rule. Facial and body hair is sparse, male sebaceous glands less active, pattern baldness, female hirsuteness and acne rare, making skin care a delightfully uncomplicated and straightforward business. Acne, operation scars or lesions may, however, appear more noticeable on coloured skins and tend to hyper-pigment, never fading entirely. Because of the normally even tone of this skin type, hyper-pigmented scars can cause illusory unevenness through troughs, pits and hollows in the skin surface. Oriental skin travels well and retains its in-built genetic inheritance, remaining as smooth and troublefree in America as in Japan. The aprocrine glands are smaller in orientals, minimising the problem of sweat and body odour, while the pigmentary anomalies that plague both white and black skins are very uncommon. Women who want to project the high-profile twentieth-century fashion look, however, start with the handicap of a 'flat canvas': a poorly defined bone structure and the narrow two-dimensional oriental eye that defies dramatic definition. Eyelid surgery to open up the eye and create a western hollow-lidded appearance remains the most popular and successful cosmetic operation to date amongst oriental women and a smaller percentage of men.

Black/Coloured Skin

If any skin has an inherent monopoly on youth, it is surely the black or coloured skin with its formidable pigmentary 'armour' that shields the deeper basal cell layer against the damaging effects of strong ultraviolet light, absorbing 30 per cent more ultraviolet light than white skins. This protection factor not only dramatically reduces the risk of skin cancer, a phenomenon more common in particularly fair white skins than any other skin type, and of sunburn and lesions due to UV damage, but confers an ageless quality on the skin keeping it smooth and supple, with minimal wrinkling and degenerative skin changes until well into the forties, fifties, and even the sixties. By which time nature's ageing signs are all to clearly etched into the white skin. Not that black skin is totally exempt from potential sun damage; as Dr Albert Kligman observes, even black skin if exposed continually and relentlessly to very harsh weather conditions and strong ultraviolet light without protection from a sun screen can develop wrinkles, lines and solar keratoses and even increase the risk of developing skin cancer.

There are over thirty-three shades of so-called black skin alone, hybrids made up of varying pigmentary permutations, a Pointilliste mêlée which can include tones ranging from aubergine, purple, and indigo to orange, yellow and ash. This explains the paucity of comprehensive and realistic make-up ranges for black and coloured skins; in particular, the dearth of natural-looking tinted foundations testifies to the heterogeneous quality of dark skin.

Some doctors think that because of a slower rate and degree of elastin degeneration, black skin withstands the ravages of sunlight and the onslaught of time not only because of its capacity to absorb ultraviolet rays, but also because in doing so it neutralises the destructive free radicals that are produced by ultra-violet light; thus there is less damage to protein and cell DNA. It is rather a long shot and he has no conclusive evidence to back him up as yet, but Dr Kligman postulates that one of the reasons why so many black men and women make naturally powerful athletes is because, he says, they have stronger, more stretchy and expandable elastin fibres. Elastin, of course, is not merely an important constituent of young-looking skin but also contributes to the elasticity of muscles, arteries, which are 40 per cent elastin, ligaments, which are 70 per cent elastin, and the suppleness of joints throughout the body. Apart from its superabundance of melanin, black skin also tends to have a sturdier constitution because of its morphology. Sweat glands are larger and more numerous in black skin, with a predominance of surface ecrine glands that keep the body cooler and more comfortable in intense heat. Because black skin allows the body to absorb more heat, the need to sweat to reduce body temperature is far greater. In the cold climates negro skins, however, react poorly. Most dermatologists agree that black skin in general contains more numerous and larger sebaceous glands which tend to be situated closer to the skin's surface, accounting for the characteristic oily, often open-pored texture of many black skins. Sebaceous secretion is often fattier and more profuse than in white skin. However, sometimes the reflection of oil on black skin, relatively unnoticeable on a white surface, accounts for its oily appearance, which is not invariably indicative of the degree of sebaceous activity. Conversely, when the surface of black skin becomes dry it assumes a dull, ashy appearance, due to the accumulation of dead skin cells that are ready to flake off. This is more apparent than on white skin, the way that marks and dust show up more on polished dark wood than, say, on pale bleached pinewood.

Against the Grain

Pseudofolliculitis — ingrown facial hairs — can prove the bane of any man past puberty who shaves regularly, but it is more of a problem amongst black men whose hair follicles are curved. The condition is directly caused by the curved hair follicle characteristic of black skin; shaving produces a sharply pointed hair that re-enters the skin. This causes a foreign-body reaction that results in abnormal scarring. Shaving initiates and aggravates the condition and the only cure is, in fact, to grow a beard, even though this may be totally unacceptable. The best treatment is to avoid using any kind of razor and opt instead for a chemical hair remover. In some cases, electrolysis of the worst affected parts of the beard may be a valuable investment in terms of aesthetics and comfort. In many men the use of depilatory products, however, can produce an irritation, and it is advisable in this case to follow the use of the depilatory with the application of lukewarm wet dressings of water rather than using soap and water. Corticosteroid creams can also be used to prevent or cure or minimise irritation.

If pigmentation and surface thickness protects black skin

against much of the damage and ageing processes common to white skin, these very features contribute a perverse debit side accounting for a genetic predisposition in particular to problems of scarring and mottled pigmentation. A major problem is that when injured, black skin in its collagen formation and repair mechanism becomes overactive, causing the formation of keloid — raised, bunched — scars in response to injury or surgical incision. Blemishes like acne scars, cuts, and lesions, as they heal, may also remain far lighter or else, quite commonly, become much more deeply pigmented than the normal surrounding skin tone and also fade more slowly and incompletely than on a white skin. This makes surgery a particular problem for those with black skins, particularly cosmetic operations to improve areas of the face and neck; even ear piercing can leave hard bulbous ridges on the earlobes of a black-skinned person. Most reputable plastic surgeons and dermatologists refuse to carry out procedures such as dermabrasion and chemical peeling, which involves removing the uppermost layers, because on dark skins it is impossible to predict whether the operation will leave scars or whether the new pigmentation will remain evenly distributed. Keloid scars — by no means exclusive to black or coloured skin — can be treated with varying degrees of success through painless injections of cortisone directly into the scar to shrink, depress and soften the hardened tissue mass. In very severe cases, the surgeon may attempt to excise the original scar, giving it a flatter contour and finer, neater outline, and follow up with steroid injections. Some plastic surgeons use pure alphatocopherol — vitamin E, known to accelerate wound healing — instead of steroids, often with excellent results.

In Africa certain tribes have long made an ornamental feature of the skin's proclivity to 'bunch' and hyper-pigment by etching patterns and markings into the face and body which form permanent and clearly defined ridges on the skin. Removal of tribal scars is something more and more westernised African women and men seek nowadays when they visit dermatologists, beauty therapists and plastic surgeons in the west. Successful cortisone treatment depends on accuracy and doses; large doses can inhibit the function of the adrenal glands which manufacture the body's own quota of cortisone, and too much injected into the surrounding tissues can cause atrophy while too much injected into the scar tissue itself can make it shiny and red. X-ray treatment is regarded by some doctors as a viable alternative if cortisone therapy fails, although others dismiss it because of the potential cancer risk.

Unless injured, black skin is no more genetically predisposed to pigmentation disorders than any other skin type — the problem is that uneven mottled pigmentation, hypo or hyper-pigmented patches alike, are far more noticeable and unaesthetic on dark than on white skins, which is why in the East a certain social stigma surrounds common and harmless skin blemishes.

Mixed Markings

The cause of vitiligo, white depigmented patches of the skin, and chloasma, dark spots and blotches, remains a mystery both in white and in dark skins alike, although the links between elevated hormone levels in pregnancy and taking the Pill and the formation of deeply pigmented facial marks and blotches is well established. Some dermatologists believe that elevated oestrogen triggers the release of a chemical called melanocyte stimulating hormone (MSH) which produces extra scattering of melanocytes. Chloasma may respond well to regular use of a hydroquinone-based bleaching cream, although the darker the natural skin colour, the greater the risk of creating an uneven mottled effect and a danger of bleaching pigment out of the surrounding area of the skin. For some years now scientists have been studying a lipophilic yeast, a fungus-caused pityriasis versicolor which causes skin pigment to scale off. If the fungus could be stabilised and synthesised in ointment form, dermatologists believe it would offer a more effective bleaching agent.

Nowhere near as serious as vitiligo patches is hypomelanosis, a common pigmentary affliction in West Indian men and women over the age of forty, which shows up as irregular pale brown dots about the size of an apple pip usually covering the trunk and limbs. Relatively inconspicuous, unlike vitilgo, these spots do not become enlarged or more unsightly, nor do they herald the early stages of vitiligo.

Often caused by a lipophilic yeast often caught on sun beds, pityriasis versicolor, which flourishes in warm, moist environments, is a common but easily treatable pigmentary disorder which affects dark and pale skinned alike, but looks worse on coloured skins. Short-term use of anti-fungal cream such as

Canestan will clear it up rapidly and completely.

Just as common but far more distressing and dreaded, both because of its effects and failure to respond to treatment, is vitiligo, suffered by about one person in a hundred and believed by many dermatologists to be an auto-immune disorder that causes small or very large areas of the skin to lose their pigmentation altogether. On brown or black skins the visual impact of vitiligo can be unsightly and deeply emotionally distressing, as the depigmented areas turn white or pale pink in a negro skin, while the unaffected skin often becomes darker, especially as a result of exposure to sunlight, throwing the demarcation line between pigmented and depigmented patches into sharper, more acute definition. Not surprisingly, the degree of disfigurement, often covering vast areas of the face, neck, chest and back, is regarded as a social stigma amongst many Asian and African communities where it is still sometimes mistakenly regarded as a symptom of a more virulent and contagious disease such as leprosy. Sadly, there is so far no cure or effective treatment for vitiligo and spontaneous remission is rare. A very small percentage of patients respond to the use of strong topical steroids on the white patches and about 20 per cent of cases are improved after lengthy photochemotherapy (PUVA treatment), which involves taking a tablet that makes the skin sensitive to strong artificial UV light and then undergoing UV radiation in an attempt to rekindle the formation of melanocytes. Unfortunately in the majority of cases, vitiligo either doesn't respond at all to PUVA therapy as it is called, or may indeed become worse as the normally pigmented areas darken and the lighter areas become mottled and speckled or only partially recover their former tone, while the edges around the white patches develop a penumbra, becoming more deeply pigmented and defined. Because of the acknowledged risk of developing cancer from prolonged UV radiation, PUVA therapy is only prescribed by doctors in very severe cases of vitiligo and especially in younger people with dark or black skins in whom the condition can prove a psychological as well as a physical disaster.

Blessing In Disguise

For those unlucky enough to suffer from severe recalcitrant hyper or hypo-pigmentary problems, the art of cosmetic camouflage, widely used amongst men and women and children with disfiguring facial birthmarks, such as port wine stains or extensive scarring, has reached a zenith of masterly perfection and realism. Although white patches are harder to disguise realistically on black compared with pale skin, the formulations, tones and nuances of these cosmetic masking creams made up of waxes, oils, pigments and the opaque covering-agent titanium dioxide, are being improved upon constantly, and there are an increasing number of beauty therapists trained in cosmetic camouflage who can advise on the right products to use and how to apply them. Referral should come from a GP, dermatologist, or a hospital; products and advice are often available on the National Health Service or via the voluntary services of the Red Cross organisation. When used on dark skins, it may be necessary to blend several colours in the camouflage make-up range to match normal skin tone, and where white patches are large or very noticeable, these should first be shaded out with an 'undercoat' darker than the normal skin tone, and then topped up with a second layer of cream to match the surrounding skin. A translucent powder is used to set the cover cream, followed by a waterproof cover cream to give a natural and lasting finish. Women can then apply their usual make-up foundation and/or powder over the complexion if and when required. So in essence camouflage make-up provides a 'second skin' upon which to build make-up effects if and as required, or to provide as nearly as possible a natural 'nude' look. Cover creams are best removed with a greasy cleansing cream, such as Crowe's Cremine; being waterproof, they cannot be shifted with soap and water alone. Practice and experimentation can ensure realistic-looking effects. Deft finger-work — patting cover creams and subtle feathery blending of various creams over the affected areas, rather than rubbing them in heavy handedly — inevitably yields a degree of coverage efficiently opaque to mask the blemishes, yet light enough not to look clown-like or chalky.

CHAPTER 8

Skin Disorders

Allergies, Eczema and Contact Dermatitis

It is estimated that over two million babies, children and adults in the UK suffer from some form of eczematous disorder sometime in their lives. The term eczema, however, is one of those vague, ambiguous words that mean so many different things to different people. Many doctors claim that skin allergies, eczema and dermatitis are all one and the same condition — an inflammation triggered by the skin's intolerance to any one of a number of hundreds of sensitising agents. But not only is this lumping together of a rag-bag of allergic symptoms into the same diagnostic basket a glib over-simplification of the whole complex nature of skin intolerance, it is also inaccurate. Eczema, atopic eczema in particular and contact dermatitis may be hard to differentiate and diagnose, but they are caused by two distinctly different mechanisms. The most vexing aspect of diagnosis lies in nailing the offending substance, because allergens are also irritants and vice versa. However, the ways in which they damage the skin can be summed up as follows:

An *allergic* skin reaction, sometimes known as allergic contact dermatitis, may result from the external application of a specific allergen as well as via the systemic absorbtion of any allergen, from house dust or cat's hair to food *to which a person may have been exposed for years without any previous sign of trouble whatever*. Whether caused by an external or internal allergen, an allergic reaction never occurs on the first contact but takes at least five to seven days to develop as a result of a massive upheaval of the body's immune system, which floods the system with massive secretions of histamine to attack the antigen in question. Symptoms can vary from an itchy red rash, scaling, blistering, rawness, flaking — classic signs of eczema — to more painful widespread symptoms, streaming and stinging eyes, swelling tissues, runny nose, swollen lips, and breathing difficulties, in fact all the trappings associated with a full-blown cell-mediated immune response. Once sensitised, the body will *always* react to *any amount* of that substance, no matter how miniscule the quantity, for the rest of that person's life. A rule that applies equally whether the allergy is caused by strawberries, shellfish, penicillin, lanolin, or a cosmetic colourant.

Atopic or *endogenous eczema* is a particularly vicious and chronic skin disorder which often develops in very young children, making their skin the target organ for disaster. The skin of atopic patients, who may also be prone to asthma and hayfever and sometimes to migraine, has an in-built defect which causes it to react adversely to a wide number of harmless substances.

The symptoms of *contact dermatitis*, also known as irritant contact dermatitis, tend usually to be to localised and identical to the above symptoms of eczema — redness, itching, etc. — but usually flare up promptly on first contact with an irritant substance if it is exceptionally harsh and/or concentrated, or else develop as a result of repeated contact with an irritant which systematically insults, weakens and erodes the skin's protective mechanism, stripping away layer upon layer of epidermal surface cells until the skin, severely damaged, develops chronic raw sores, cracking, peeling, etc. The hands are the commonest site for the development of cosmetic dermatitis, because they are constantly exposed to irritant substances. Contrary to an allergy, the development of contact dermatitis is dependent on the concentration or period of application of the surface. Brief exposure to a weaker concentration of an irritant substance which years previously may have caused skin damage does not necessarily mean that the damage will automatically recur.

On the Alert

It is one of the quirks of sod's law governing skin disease that the boundaries between allergy and contact dermatitis, although theoretically well defined, can even to the medical eye become blurred and confusing, since irritants and allergens can work synergistically, one potentiating the effects of the other. The corrosive effects of a detergent soap, for example, may irritate the epidermal barrier and impair its natural defences, thereby triggering the onset of an allergic reaction to a perfume or cosmetic colouring agent. A chemical molecule can prove caustic in high doses or a potential allergen in low doses.

The scale of skin 'intolerance' is a broad one encompassing viciously acute or chronic damage and the discomfort of allergies, eczema and contact dermatitis at one end, to minor transient stinging, redness, smarting, and symptomatic irritation at the other. Approximately 3 to 9 per cent of the population of the UK suffer an adverse reaction to a cosmetic or toiletry product in any one year. Two to six per cent of these are likely to be irritant in nature, and only about 1 per cent or possibly less represent an allergic reaction. Women often complain of 'being allergic' to certain brands of cosmetics when, in fact, they are merely sensitive to and prone to irritation by some of the ingredients. Maddeningly, there is no rule of thumb as far as choosing a failsafe brand. In general, the more fair, dry and delicate the skin, the more likely it is to prove intolerant to a wide range of cosmetic toiletries including soap and shampoo, which are harsh by nature, although hypo-allergenic products, commonly fragrance-free and formulated with a minimum amount of known potential allergens and irritant substances, are in general kinder to touchy skin. Given the vast battery of synthetic and natural ingredients used in modern cosmetics — at the last count not less than 5,000 different substances were listed by the American Cosmetics, Toiletries and Fragrance Association Dictionary — it is somewhat amazing that there aren't more reported cases of cosmetic irritation and allergy. As it stands, the most any manufacture of hypo-allergenic products can do is drastically reduce the amount of raw materials. The French company Roc, for example, use a maximum of 170 substances as opposed to the figure of roughly 1,000 ingredients incorporated into products manufactured by the large multi-national cosmetic companies. Fragrance is a major offender, composed as it often is of as many as a hundred different constituents, as are colouring agents of which, for example, eosin and its derivatives, chromium fillers, cobalt blues, and pearlising agents are recognised for their irritant and allergic properties. Out of about 160 commonly used colouring agents, a bare dozen or so may prove innocuous enough to include in a reputable hypo-allergenic make-up range.

Gums, alginates, sulfamides, preservatives such as formalde-hyde, oils and emollients including lanolin, and alcohol make up the remaining suspect ingredients whose use is generally restricted or eliminated altogether in the manufacture of more bland and gentle cosmetics.

Nevertheless, stringency notwithstanding, the term hypo-allergenic is often misconstrued as a guarantee of total safety for every user, when all it merely indicates is that any given product is *less* likely to cause allergy or irritation, although it is worth bearing in mind that the degree of allergen exclusion varies from company to company. Since skin irritation flares up almost immediately, it is normally an easy matter to nail the offender and stop using the product, giving a clear-cut solution to the problem.

Detection

Potential irritants with which we routinely bombard ourselves through our hobbies, housework, toiletry, and occupation, by the clothes we wear, let alone the food we eat and the environment we live in, have risen by leaps and bounds over the past few decades, so that dermatologists often have the devil's own work to root out the correct allergen or contact sensitiser in any given case of contact dermatitis or allergy. Patch testing and monitoring of a person's lifestyle can help. Soaps, detergents, household cleansers, glues, resins, and rubber are common everyday household irritants responsible for a large percentage of eczema-tous problems suffered, for example, by women who spend long periods with their hands immersed in water, bleach, soaps and detergents. Often simply wearing cotton-lined rubber gloves to protect the skin is all that is needed to cure the condition. Some people, on the other hand, may be impervious to detergents yet prove allergic to rubber, a recognised sensitiser. Certainly the most important single step towards curing or controlling irritant or allergic contact dermatitis (CD) is to avoid wherever possible all contact with the offending substance or group of irritants — more easily said than done in the case of occupational or so-called industrial dermatitis, where, unless proper precautions to protect the skin are taken, the choice may consist of redundancy, finding alternative employment, or continuing to suffer discomfort and disfigurement. Occupational dermatitis (OD) comprises 60–65 per cent of all occupational diseases, making up 50 per cent of all cases of dermatitis seen by doctors, and it accounts not only for widespread misery and suffering but for a significant financial loss to industry generally. Given free rein, the harsh chemicals responsible for inducing irritant CD will completely wear down the skin's resistance and destroy its top layers, heaping repeated insult upon injury and causing excessive and chronic dryness, cracking, crusting, blisters, flaking, weeping, and soggy patches of skin tissue as fluid collects and seeps through the damaged surface; infection by bacteria and the formation of abscesses or pustules further complicates the condition and makes it more distressing and uncomfortable. All symptoms are, of course, greatly exacerbated — or even caused — by self-inflicted damage through repeated vigorous scratching. All allergic and irritant skin conditions are fiendishly itchy. To a degree, therefore, severe eczema is a state of cause and effect. Priority number one, along with protecting the skin against the offending substances, it to avoid the use of soap and water, opting instead for an emulsifying ointment to cleanse the skin, such as Aqueous Cream BP, an over-the-counter product which can also be used as an emollient cream throughout the day to soften the skin's surface, restore its destroying protective mechanism, and reduce itchiness. Other bland, healing soothing creams are Boots E45 cream and Eczederm Cream, which can also be used throughout the day. Since water can be calculated upon to dry out skin even further, adding a softening substance such as Emulsifying Ointment BP into the bath can help to minimise the drying effects of bathing. Cold water compresses applied to the worst affected areas will help to sooth discomfort, eliminate itchiness and help healing, and anti-histamine tablets can also be taken to relieve itchiness especially during the night, when sufferers are more likely to scratch the skin and unknowingly create further damage. Many doctors prescribe either short or long-term therapy with corticosteroid creams or ointment as, for instance, Betnovate or Synalar for very stubborn and severe cases. There is little doubt that these can control and heal all forms of irritation and allergy very successfully, relieving both the discomfort and unsightliness associated with all forms of eczema. However, a word of caution. The price paid for relief gained from these potent steroid skin drugs can prove unacceptably high. In recent years tremendous controversy has risen as to the use of steroid ointments in all but the most severe and disabling cases of eczema, since they are known to cause thinning, reddening and atrophy of the skin by damaging and breaking up its collagen infrastructure, causing stretch marks and excessive sensitisation to ultraviolet light and extremes of hot, cold and dry atmospheres. Worse, the skin can get 'hooked' on corticosteroids, temporary improvement giving way to a horrific rebound eczema and a flare up of former symptoms or worse once therapy is stopped. In very strong doses, they can suppress the function of the adrenal glands and undermine the immune defence system, the body's disease-fighting surveillance and detection system. Undoubtedly steroid creams have their place, correctly prescribed and monitored by a GP or dermatologist, but they must *only* be used on the affected patches of skin, if possible never on the face or on or around the eyes, and they must on no account be lent out to friends or family as one might an ordinary, innocuous, over-the-counter skin preparation, since they can prove as powerful and therefore as hazardous as any internal medicine.

Trials of the Trade

Contact dermatitis of either variety can occur at any age from eight to eighty and may be caused through very gradual, insidious sensitisation to one commonly used substance such as a favourite lipstick, soap or hand cream over a period of many years. Sometimes it may take extreme heat, cold, dry or humid atmospheres, ultraviolet light or the use of drugs to act as a catalyst in triggering the actual mechanism of the skin eruption, so it is no use being complacent about eczema — just because you have never had it doesn't mean you can't eventually develop it from a substance that you have been using for many years. Sometimes the actual site of a rash or eruption is misleading — redness or swelling of the eyelid, for instance, is commonly traced to nail varnish or hand cream, which often comes into contact with the eyes only during the night when a person touches their face while asleep. Certain drugs can also cause photo-allergy or photo-sensitivity, setting off a rash, swelling or patchy pigmentation on exposure to strong sunlight and the UV rays used in sunbeds. Antibiotics (sulphonamides and tetracyclines), anti-fungal agents, diuretics and some psychotropic drugs (anti-depressants, tranquillisers) are the main offenders. In Britain and the rest of Europe and America, there is a standard patch test that includes the twenty-three most common allergic sensitisers to which other suspected substances are added if primary testing yields no clues. But be prepared sometimes for a long and arduous search for the precise bogey that is causing all the trouble.

Commonly acknowledged sensitisers almost everyone comes into daily contact with are all harsh, abrasive cleaners — soaps, detergents, bleach, washing-up liquid — nylon and other man-made fibres and lanolin present in a vast array of products, plastic, resins as used in glue, nickel and metal used in zips, bra fasteners and watch-straps, rubber, rubber additives like latex used in gloves, girdles, bras and even contraceptive sheaths! Hair-removers, anti-perspirants and sundry toiletry items, hair dyes and colourants, are in particular a well-known and very powerful contact irritant. This still leaves the formidable battery of sensitisers found in cases of so-called industrial dermatitis, the chemicals indigenous to each specific trade or profession.

HAZARDS OF COMMON OCCUPATIONS

1. *Dentists, dental technicians and dental nurses*

Allergens	Local anaesthetics
	Metal alloys (e.g mercury)
	Antibiotics
	Perfumes (essential oils of cloves eugenol, spearmint and cinnamon
	Plastics — often acrylic
	Natural waxes
	Colophony (rosin)
	Rubber gloves
	Dental impression material
Irritants	Water
	Disinfectants
	Soaps
	X-rays

2. *Electricians, electronics workers*

Allergens	Welding fluxes
	Epoxy and phenol formaldehyde re-sins
	Rubber
	Colophony
Irritants	Soldering fluxes
	Solvents

3. *Engineers*

Allergens	Welding fluxes
	Resins
	Rubber
Allergens and Irritants	Adhesives
	Paints
Irritants	Oils of many types
	Solvents and cleaning fluids

4. *Bakers, confectioners and cooks*

Allergens	Benzyl peroxide
	Ammonium persulphate
Allergens and Irritants	Spices and flavouring agents
	Nut oils
	Fruits
	Vegetables
Irritants	Water
	Soaps
	Detergents
	Flour
Miscellaneous	Mites in flour

5.   *Hairdressers and barbers*

Allergens	Dyes
	Perfumes
	A range of cosmetic sensitisers
	Metals
	Rubber
	Preservatives
Irritants	Water
	Detergents
	Soaps
	Shampoos
	Perm lotion
	Bleaches

6.   *Builders, masons, etc.*

Allergens	Chromates
	Epoxy resins
	Phenolic resins
Irritants	Alkalis (limes)
	Water
	Abrasives
	Fibre glass

7.   *Carpenters, wood machinists and cabinet makers*

Allergens	Epoxy resins
	Perfumes (used in polishes)
	Glues
Allergens and Irritants	Sawdust from woods used
	Stains, paints and varnishes
	Wood preservatives
Irritants	Solvents/thinners
	Linseed oil

8. *Office workers*

Allergens   Glues
                        Metals (especially nickel)
                        Rubber
                        Duplicating paper

Irritants   Low humidity environment
                           (the air-conditioned office)
                        Solvents
                        Soap
                        Photocopying (ammonia)

9. *Florists, horticulturalists and gardeners*

Allergens   Woods
                        Lichens

Allergens and   Plants
Irritants   Fungicides, herbicides and insecti-
                           cides

Irritants   Water

10. *Beauty therapists, manicurists and masseurs*

Allergens   Ingredients of beauty creams and lo-
                           tions
                        Perfumes
                        Preservatives and antimicrobials
                        Waxes
                        Lanolin
                        Dyes (in hair dyes)
                        Artificial fingernails
                        Resins
                        Adhesives

Allergens and   Shampoo
Irritants

Irritants
Water
Soap
Disinfectants
Alcohol (used as a solvent for oils and as a cleanser)
Ultraviolet light

11. *Photographers*

Allergens
Rubber (gloves)

Allergens and Irritants
Developers
Fixers
Hardeners
Intensifiers (hydroquinone)
Toners
Colour developers

Irritants
Water
Solvents
Tray cleaners

12. *Physicians and nurses*

Allergens
Medicaments, e.g.:–
  antibiotics
  anaesthetics   } topical
  antihistamines
Rubber gloves

Allergens and Irritants
Disinfectants and germicides

Irritants
Water
Soap and detergents

13. *Workers in the rubber industry*

    Allergens   Accelerators
                                   Antioxidants
                                   Plasticisers
                                   Dyes

    Irritants   Solvents
                                   Soaps and detergents

14. *Agricultural workers*

    Allergens   Antibiotic food additives
                                   Medicaments
                                   Rubber (clothing)

    Allergens and   Antiseptics and disinfectants
    Irritants   Oils (petrol and diesel)
                                   Wood preservatives
                                   Plants

    Irritants   Insecticides, fungicides and herbicides
                                   Paints
                                   Solvents
                                   Detergents
                                   Water

15. *Animal laboratory workers and veterinary surgeons*

    Allergens   Medicaments
                                   Rubber gloves

    Allergens and   Antiseptics and disinfectants
    Irritants

    Irritants   Soaps and detergents
                                   Water

    Miscellaneous   Microbial infections
                                   Contact urticaria from animal tissues

Thoughts and Theories

Just why certain substances are tolerated by millions of people yet cause untold misery in certain unfortunate individuals has puzzled dermatologists for decades. However, specialists in the allied field of immunology and clinical ecology studying the cause and effect mechanism of such related disorders as asthma, hay fever, migraine and chronic atopic eczema, may well uncover vital clues as to the idiosyncrasies of unhealthy skin. Atopic eczema — very common in babies and young children as well as adults, and often accompanied by asthma and respiratory problems — appears to be caused by an inherited defect in the body's immune defence system, causing a massive allergic reaction to a wide variety of external allergens — foods, household dust, feathers, mites, animal hairs, pollen, and a myriad of other everyday environmental contaminants. An abnormal immune response to such normally harmless antigens, in particular the tendency for the body to manufacture excessive amounts of what are called IgE antibodies is, speculate immunologists, probably one of the principle characteristics of these atopic individuals prone to wheezing, weeping, swelling and eczema at the drop of a cat's hair!

The immunopathological theory of atopic eczema has gained credibility with the discovery that sufferers also appear more prone to the development of smallpox, cowpox and herpes viruses, and suffer recurrent bacterial infections. Breast feeding may well confer protection against atopic eczema and allergies in general by strengthening and building up a healthy immune system at the earliest age possible. At the Hospital for Sick Children in London, studies aimed at reducing the incidents of atopic eczema in children of atopic parents show that babies who are breast-fed for as long as possible, avoiding common allergens such as cow's milk and other dairy produce, have a lower instance of eczema than bottle-fed babies. It has also been known for quite some years that children with atopic eczema have reduced blood levels of unsaturated fatty acids, which explains why oil of evening primrose, a rich source of linoleic and gamma-linoleic acid, seems to produce a small but significant amount of improvement in patients with atopic eczema. Oil of evening primrose is marketed under the brand-name of Efamol, and the daily dosage thought to be sufficient to help people suffering from eczema is 500 mg a day.

Cysts and Boils

Frequently confused, the two are nevertheless quite different in structure and usually in appearance. Boils may form on otherwise unblemished healthy skin, though they tend to feature more commonly as a part of acne, especially on the face and neck and particularly under tight shirt collars around a man's beard area, on the buttocks and the arms, forming as an abscess within infected hair follicles. This explains their livid appearance and extreme tenderness. As a boil matures, it produces a postular 'head' which may burst and leave a pitted scar. By comparison, a cyst is relatively benign, a non-inflamed smooth sac-like structure that is lined with a layer of skin-like material. It may begin either as a plugged gland or build up as a result of pieces of skin piling up and becoming buried beneath the surface. Only if a cyst becomes infected and inflamed or ruptures does it resemble a boil. If it doesn't disappear, a cyst can be simply removed through either cryo therapy — freezing of the skin with either liquid nitrogen or carbon dioxide — or electro-desiccation — 'zapping' of the skin with a hair-thin electro-surgical needle which singes the target area.

Boils present a somewhat trickier challenge, especially if they are a recurrent problem. The simplest solution is to lance the abscess, incising it to promote drainage. Washing the infected area with a hexachlorophene-based anti-bacterial solution such as pHiso-med helps to prevent the spread of infection, and the application of warm compresses can accelerate the maturation of an abscess. Meticulous personal hygiene, showering and bathing frequently and changing bed linen and underwear regularly is essential. Squeezing must be avoided at all costs, since this is bound to spread the infection. In the case of very stubborn and/or recurrent boils, antibiotics may be prescribed to control the infection. Some chronic sufferers may be tested for diabetes, in which there is a predisposition for the development of boils.

Warts

Possibly the commonest of all skin afflictions, warts rate high among the enigmas of modern medicine. Their resistance makes them the bane of any dermatologist's life. Fundamentally just a hardened, impacted, overgrowth of keratinised skin cells with a raised edge and a rough surface, these are caused by a human wart virus and are therefore contagious, though totally harmless. There are about twelve different wart viruses depending on where they appear; genital warts, for example, differ from plantar warts or verrucas, which form on the soles of the feet, and these may vary again from facial or finger warts. They tend to be commonest in children and teenagers and often disappear spontaneously, and immunity seems to develop with age, preventing their subsequent reappearance. The life-cycle of warts seems to be determined by their own inner timetable, which is totally unpredictable and erratic. Verrucas are particularly tenacious and uncomfortable because the pressure of walking pushes them inwards and sideways, often squeezing the nerve endings as a result. Pressure, friction or damage to the skin may encourage the spread of warts, which explains why chronic nail-biters are often afflicted, making ragged fingertips look even more unsightly than usual. Verrucas are notoriously stubborn to treat and may need a series of treatments to cut out, burn or freeze off the growths, using either a scalpel, a strong caustic solution, liquid nitrogen, electro-surgical desiccation, or even a carbon-dioxide laser, the fastest, most painless method of removing warts.

The dermatologist's challenge lies in destroying every last cell deep within the growth; failure to do so means that if the living virus still remains, the wart will re-establish itself. Genital warts affecting the penis and the vulva are on the increase, according to neurologists, and are highly contagious and need prompt medical attention. One or two applications of podopholin or trichloracetic acid work fairly promptly in removing genital warts. Those that do not respond can be quickly and painlessly vapourised with a carbon-dioxide laser or painted with a potent drug, 5-Fluorouracil, often used for skin cancers. If in doubt or embarrassed about genital warts, a visit to the Genito-Urinary Medical Department of any large hospital offers the fastest, most accurate diagnosis and the chance of the most expert medical attention. A dermatologist is the best person to tackle facial warts safely without risk of skin damage, while there are a number of tried and tested over-the-counter wart cures containing salicylic acid which can be used on other parts of the body. These include

Avrogel, Ayrtons Corn and Wart Paint, Salactol, and Wartex Ointment. These preparations will need to be applied to the warts for a few weeks or months before they disappear, either temporarily or permanently. They must *never* be used on the face or genital areas.

Hope for sufferers lies in the wizardry of genetic engineering. Scientists hope that by identifying the DNA structure of the different wart viruses it should eventually be possible to develop an anti-viral drug or a vaccine to stimulate the body's immunity to the wart virus. In fact there is some research that suggests that interferon, a chemical produced by the body to combat infections which has recently been studied as a cancer fighter in synthetic form, may also one day prove a weapon against the most resistant of genital warts. Studies at the Duke University Medical Centre show that over 70 per cent of patients with genital warts that were unresponsive to other treatment were healed by repeated injections of interferon.

Rather different in appearance to the common or garden wart are the dark, flat, rough-textured seborrhoeic or senile warts which develop from late middle age onwards, generally on the torso, increasing in size and shape with age to the point where one mark can sometimes cover large areas of skin or else smaller ones can develop by the hundreds. Sometimes mistaken for malignant moles, seborrhoeic warts are entirely benign and not connected with sunlight. They can be surgically removed if they prove embarrassing or unsightly.

Moles

Basically a highly concentrated area of pigment cells, the average adult usually has dozens of moles of varying sizes dotted all over the face and body — in the majority of cases all totally benign and thus harmless. Moles that are large, prominent and generally unaesthetic can be removed easily enough by freezing with liquid nitrogen, electro-surgical desiccation, or even laser treatment, leaving no or minimal scarring and without in any way risking the development of malignancy. Dermatologists, however, quite rightly prefer to err on the side of caution if a mole, or any blemish or lesion for that matter, looks in the least irregular or suspicious, as this could well portend malignancy and a premalignant growth. It is worth pointing out, however, that the chance of a common 'regular' mole proving malignant tends to be about one in a million. However, should you notice any of the following changes, no matter how minor, in a pre-existing mole, you must seek medical advice without delay.

*Any change of colour, especially mottling or patchy areas of black, brown, red, blue.

*Any change in shape including flattening of the surface, indentations, and loss of the smooth circular contour that distinguishes a benign mole.

*Bleeding.

*The formation of miniscule pinpoint moles around the periphery of a pre-existing one.

*Any increases in size.

*Any pain, tenderness or itching.

*Formation of a new mole where previously none existed.

Never, never prick, squeeze, or rub a mole — it could be quite literally fatal; nor procrastinate: the difference between seeing a specialist within a few days or a few weeks could quite simply turn out to be a matter of life and death. If a specialist is at all suspicious, he will arrange to have a biopsy taken to establish whether a mole is benign or whether, as in only about 20 per cent of cases of patients who report a 'suspicious' mole, it is malignant. In which case if it were allowed to develop untreated, this proves the deadliest of all skin cancers. A five-year survival rate from malignant melanoma as it is called is no more than approximately 30 per cent. The majority of melanomas, however, do develop on normal healthy skin — even on areas not exposed to sunshine such as the buttocks — and as such are, in theory at any rate, easy enough to detect in the very early stages when they can still be removed and successfully treated, via chemotherapy, radiation or excision, depending at what stage the cancer has been discovered.

Other Cancerous and Pre-cancerous Disorders

These include principally rodent ulcers and solar or actinic keratoses more likely to occur after the age of forty-five or fifty-five than in youth. These are a direct, obvious and cumulative result of sun-damaged skin and are twice as common in men than in women. The links between excessive exposure to sunlight and skin cancer are by now truly established beyond any shadow of a doubt, and not surprisingly therefore the fair, freckly, Celtic skin, especially of those people living in hot sunny climates and working out of doors, is most likely to fall victim to some form of skin cancer. Mass immigration of men and women with fair colouring to countries like Australia and South Africa, increased leisure time and outdoor hobbies, holidays in hot sunny climates, the fashion for suntanning, have all contributed to the appalling increase in skin cancer which today constitutes one out of every four cancers. Solar keratoses though initially benign are usually regarded as the most widespread precursor to skin cancer and appear as red or pink scaly plaques, gritty or rough to the touch and sometimes mistaken for psoriasis or ringworm. Whilst in a harmless, benign state, solar keratoses can quite easily be removed through Cryosurgery, electro-surgical desiccation, laser treatment or dermabrasion, in order to prevent deterioration. Adopting a complacent wait and see attitude when these blemishes appear is not only foolish and shortsighted, it could prove tantamount to signing a death warrant. Changes in sun-damaged skin that bode serious trouble are mainly increased scaliness and redness, the formation of a lump or crust on existing patches which, on shedding, exposes a raised nodule, any bleeding from a pre-existing lump or blemish, or the appearance of a persistent wound which refuses to heal. Any of these must be medically diagnosed and if necessary a small patch of tissue tested for malignancy. Though solar keratoses can appear singly, they are more likely to form in groups of four to twelve and most vulnerable sites are the ears, eyes, lips, forearms, hands and forehead, areas commonly 'caught' repeatedly by the sun. When diagnosed early enough, these malignant patches can be removed and treated, usually with 100 per cent success, either through excision, radiation, or the use of powerful cancer-killing drugs including one of the retinoic acids similar to those used to treat acne and psoriasis. Unlike other forms of cancer the prognosis on these types of malignant tumours is generally good, since they do not metastasise (i.e. spread to other parts of the body). Only 2 to 10 per cent of skin cancers ever spread to the internal organs and tissues, and conversely internal cancers almost never spread to the skin. Common too in people who burn easily in the sun is another form of malignant tumour called a rodent ulcer, which generally appears on the face as a shiny nodule (in its initial stage of development it can be as small as an eighth of an inch in diameter with tiny blood vessels crossing its surface), which eventually ulcerates and refuses to heal. If promptly treated, their growth can be arrested and the malignancy destroyed with minimal scarring or risk of it spreading to other areas of skin.

Because pre-cancerous changes in the skin are so readily detectable and therefore treatable in the very early stages, it is impossible to over emphasise the importance of keeping tabs on any blemishes, lumps, bumps and irregularities that might appear on the face and body and seeking medical advice if any of these seem in the least bit suspicious. The more you expose your skin to sunlight and the elements in general, the more vigilant and hawk-eyed should be your attitude to your skin whether you are male or female. No matter how small and insignificant a skin lesion may seem, no GP or dermatologist in their right mind will regard you as neurotic or alarmist for arranging a consultation at the earliest possible opportunity to rule out the possibility of malignancy. Quite the contrary. Unlike *every other form of malignancy*, skin cancer stands out as the one variety which can be easily identified in its earlier stages and usually reponds with a 100 per cent success to prompt treatment. Thus the alarming rise in past decades in the rate of skin cancer directly due to sun damage, fully justifies regular expert vigilance and surveillance as a fundamental life-saving precaution. The other priority is of course avoiding the sun damage that precipitates these degenerative changes in the first place, of which more in another chapter.

If failure or a delay in seeing a doctor can cost you your life, then just as disastrous can be the temptation to take matters, quite literally, into your own hands. While the folly of picking and squeezing acne lesions, for example, is all too amply and evidently recorded in the scars and pits that mar the complexions of millions of adults the world over, the consequences of tampering with an isolated, persistent ulcer, mole or blemish can prove fatal. Dermatologists are constantly sounding off about our seemingly masochistic delight in self-mutilation and the irresistible compulsion to pluck, pick, scratch, squeeze and generally aggravate any protuberance or irregularity that forms on the skin's surface. This habit in some people — especially when under stress or suffering from nervous tension — can, like nail biting, for example, become subconsious, totally obsessive, and ultimately lead to horrendous repercussions, opening up a Pandora's box of self-induced skin ailments. The two cardinal rules in all skin eruptions are *don't touch* and, when in doubt, *consult your doctor immediately.*

Capillary Disorders

Rosacea

The medical term acne rosacea is a confusing one, since this is a chronic hyper-sensitivity of the face which bears no relationship whatever to the greasiness and pore problems of acne vulgaris, other than the appearance of tiny pinhead pimples or purplish lumps beneath the skin's surface. Characterised by sporadic outbreaks or a perpetual state of violent flushing or acute redness of the face, often accompanied by swelling, bumps, lumps, and broken veins, rosacea usually develops in middle age and its cause remains unknown. Rosacea is invariably aggravated by extremes of temperature, sunlight (sufferers must take every precaution to avoid undue exposure to strong UV light), alcohol, very hot drinks and spicy foods, and emotional stress. In short, anything which causes the already congested and weakened blood vessels of the face to dilate even further, and the skin's sensitive surface to become irritated and inflamed. Unfortunately little can be done to treat the condition successfully. Avoiding all aggravating factors, using a bland soothing skin cream and hypo-allergenic cosmetics helps to keep redness and irritation under control, while camouflage or a green tinted foundation cream can 'cool' flushed cheeks and hide very noticeable broken red veins. Provided they are not too extensive, broken capillaries can be removed through electrolysis, although some therapists may dissuade against treatment since it has a mildly irritant effect in itself. In very severe cases, where rosacea is accompanied by a rash of tiny pustules and bumps, a long-term course of tetracycline therapy may at least control this aspect of the disorder —

although, as with acne, when treatment is stopped the spots may reappear, triggered by a vigorous rebound action. A recent study conducted at Glasgow Royal Infirmary shows that isotretinoin — a potent synthetic vitamin-A derivative used to treat psoriasis — may reduce the number of pustular lesions sometimes accompanying rosacea, although the high number of possible side effects associated with the drug hardly makes it a viable first choice of treatment. Iatrogenic rosacea (i.e. therapy-induced rosacea) is technically a rosacea-like dermatitis which can occur when either psoriasis or eczema sufferers have undergone prolonged therapy with a fluorinated corticosteroid ointment on the face and then stopped using the ointment, with the result that the now sensitised, thinned and fragile skin sometimes becomes red and flushed, burns, becomes spotty, lumpy and swollen, and the capillary walls, weakened by the action of the steroid, rupture and cause flushing of the face.

Rhinophyma

Often the object of much derision and embarrassment, depending on which way you view it, is the grotesquely bulbous, red or purple-veined, so-called drinker's nose, a chronic affliction of Rabelaisian proportions which affects mainly middle-aged and older men, but is very rare in women. A severe, localised form of rosacea, it is no reflection on a person's alcoholic intake although, as in the case of all problems involving superficial blood vessels, alcohol, tea, coffee, and very hot and highly spiced foods can exacerbate the condition. There are theories that rhinophyma and rosacea may both be caused by either a disorder within the lining of the stomach and intestines, by an allergy, or else by a parasite that affects the skin's follicles, causing the lumpiness and leatheriness, but so far there is no evidence to support any of these theories. Apart from electrolysis to remove large broken veins, there is no cure for the condition other than plastic surgery to plane or slice away the misshapen, superfluous, lumpy areas of flesh and re-chisel the fleshy tissue to give near perfect proportions. Large doses of retinoic acid (synthetic vitamin A) taken internally can sometimes help to control and reduce the condition. Although it sounds simple enough in theory, unlike a regular nose job which remodels the structure of the nose from within, the external procedure can leave a certain amount of unattractive scar tissue unless a fine skin graft is taken from another part of the body. However, to many sufferers scars may prove a small price to pay for trading a nose of caricature for one of character.

Broken Veins (Telangiectases)

Broken veins are by comparison a relatively minor cosmetic problem caused by excessively dilated and thus more noticeable capillaries whose walls have become weakened and sometimes ruptured. It is a problem tha can occur at any age and affect every skin type, not just dry or delicate skin as is popularly supposed. Usually these red spidery streaks are most prominent on the cheeks, bridge and sides of the nose, under the eyes where the facial skin is thinnest, and on the legs, where they tend to be more bluish, profuse and bruise-like, and portend varicose veins or circulatory problems. They have a multitude of possible causes or combination of causes including excessive sun damage, exposure to extreme hard weather conditions, drinking alcohol, very hot tea and coffee, eating spicy food, high blood pressure, and the use of topical steroid ointments. Broken capillaries appear as a result of the weakening of the vessel walls, allowing them to rupture and leak into the surface tissues. Facial veins if not too profuse can be disguised very effectively with a special concealer stick, like Max Factor's Erase or Clinique's Quick Corrector, or, if more pronounced, with camouflage make-up. Fine broken thread veins can be successfully removed or reduced in number by one or two well-established methods such as electrolysis, where a fine needle powered by a short-wave current is used to cauterise the blood vessels, blocking off the flow of blood. Up to two or three sessions may be needed, depending on the extent of veins to be treated, to treat the mark successfully. Painless except for a mild, prickling or tickling sensation, the skin swells up for a couple of days and scabs may form where the needle is inserted. To avoid scarring these must not be picked off. More severe broken veins including the deeper bluish ones on the leg can be treated with scleotherapy. Scleotherapy involves minute injections of a chemical sclerosing fluid that collapses and closes up the inner tube of the offending vessels allowing the escaped traces of blood to dry out and fade away as the broken capillary wall is sealed off. An increasing number of dermatologists and plastic surgeons are now beginning to use a carbon-dioxide laser beam to cauterise broken veins in a few seconds without discomfort, bleeding or risk of skin damage.

Port Wine Stains

Red coloured birthmarks can, according to their size and location, prove the most horrendously traumatic affliction suffered by men and women alike. Until recently, the only method of minimising their appearance or 'shock value' was by the application of special heavy camouflage make-up, but recently, reports of successful fading of the birthmarks as a result of laser therapy have inspired hopes in the hearts of millions and millions of sufferers the world over. It is vital to emphasise however, that laser therapy for port wine stains is just emerging from its research and early experimental stages and is by no means effective in all cases. Some patients respond very well with persistent lightening of the stains but others fail to show any improvement whatsoever. What is more, it is impossible to tell who will and who will not prove to be a good candidate for treatment. Laser treatment, however, does constitute a tremendous breakthrough in the treatment of birthmarks which were once almost untreatable. They are a mass of blood vessels and being red absorb the blue/green light of the argon laser beam. This light, which can only be absorbed by the colour red, is passed through the pale layers of the skin to the network of red cells which make up the port wine stain. There it heats the blood, causing it to clot, seal and eventually be replaced by white tissue. Not only are the effects, however, not guaranteed, but there has to be a preliminary patch test which in fact is a window on the whole thing, followed by six-months waiting period to determine how much blanching if any there is of the red area. Adults over the age of about thirty or thirty-five respond best of all because the blood vessels which make up the stain get bigger with age and they proliferate more and rise up to the surface of the skin, allowing the laser light to reach them more easily. There is, for obvious reasons, a very long waiting list to date of desperate people waiting for laser treatment, despite the fact that laser therapy can only be obtained in a few specialised units in hospitals in Britain and treatment is largely in an experimental stage. It is also an expensive treatment if undertaken on a private basis, and only those people suffering from very severe disfigurement would succeed in receiving treatment on the NHS. Though if correctly administered by a trained surgeon there should be absolutely no risk of pain or scarring or damage to the tissues, there does, however, remain a very real danger that if given by an untrained practitioner unfamiliar with the use of the laser beam in skin disorders, sometimes quite extensive scarring can occur through misuse of the beam.

Excess Facial/Body Hair

Distribution and degree of body hair in a woman is largely dictated by heredity and hormones. Relatively profuse body hair where, for example, hair grows between the breasts, where the bikini line extends from the pubic area to cover large areas of the abdomen and thighs, and facial hair that is coarse and strong say on the upper lip and the chin, is inevitably due to extra high levels of the male sex hormone testosterone circulating in the body. Only if excess hair is accompanied by a deep voice, under-developed breasts, lack of periods and sexual characteristics such as, say, an enlarged clitoris, is this a sign of *abnormally* high hormonal imbalance. Excess hair may also be a sign of an ovarian or adrenal gland tumour or be caused by certain drugs. Compared to the northern countries women from southern Mediterranean climates and parts of Asia, for example, tend often to have more facial and body hair since this frequently still symbolises femininity and sexual attractiveness. As in centuries gone by, when Roman women assiduously removed every vestige of body hair by a variety of methods, and the early Greeks according to Aristophanes followed the vogue for a clean-shaven pubic area to increase their appeal to the opposite sex, the demand for temporary or permanent removal of superfluous facial and body hair remains as popular in the west as ever. The smooth 'natural look' is now well established, and increased leisure time and longer holidays generally mean more time spent wearing revealing dresses, bikinis and swimsuits. Women are therefore increasingly conscious and intolerant of unattractive surplus hair. Basically the hair-growth cycle determines how easily, rapidly and permanently hair may be removed. The cycle consists of the anagen growing stage which is accompanied by a lot of cellular division around the base of the follicle. Hair removed at this stage is more likely to grow back after six to eight weeks due to cellular activity in the matrix area. Next is the catagen transition stage: as the hair is being removed, the root forms into a club or brush-shaped end. The existing hair travels up the follicle and is shed naturally. The follicle atrophies, becomes shallow and withers up into a superficial structure. This is the weakest point of the growth cycle and hairs epilated at that stage should be permanently destroyed. Last is the telogen or resting stage: the follicle waits until a new hair is formed and is not active at the base. Cellular division propagates the whole cycle again and a new fine hair emerges from the follicle. In healthy hair-growth this stage may be transitory, with hairs being replaced immediately, a common cause of confusion in epilation; the original hair is removed and another new hair emerges from the same follicle!

Electrolysis is still regarded by most people in the beauty profession as the most efficient and proven method of permanent hair removal. There are two main types of electrolysis used in salons today: the direct current or galvanism, involving chemical destruction of the papilla which continues after a fine needle has introduced the initial negative pole of the current into the tissues, and the high frequency current or diathermy, where a fine needle is inserted into the follicle, a mild current is applied for a fraction of a second which coagulates the papilla, and the reaction ceases when the current is switched off. The loosened hair is gently lifted out with a pair of tweezers. Although less permanent than the galvanic current, this method destroys the papilla more quickly. Only a mild tingling should be felt as the current is applied. Any irritation and redness or swelling disappears within a few hours, although some people with sensitive skins may experience a crusting over of the area, but there should be no scarring if the hair removal is expertly carried out. Gradually hair-growth is discouraged with each treatment, although delay occurs if hair has previously been plucked, shaved or waxed as the follicle becomes twisted and distorted and the root and papilla more deeply imbedded. Curved follicles, on face or body, are also notoriously resistant to treatment.

There is a relatively new concept in hair removal which has revolutionised conventional methods of electrolysis. This is called the tweezer method, is marketed under the trade name of Depilex, and works on the principle of using the hair as a conducting agent. A continuous supply of radio frequency is applied through the tweezers which grip the hair, and after several seconds the shrivelled hair is gently removed. As the tweezers never come into contact with the skin there is no discomfort and no risk of scarring. A lotion is used to moisten the hairs, as there is generally insufficient natural moisture in the hair to act as a conductor for the electrical charge. Although the manufacturers do not claim that this method is permanent, they say that painless destruction of the hair is progressively achieved, but controversy still surrounds the tweezer method and centres around the argument that there isn't sufficient moisture in the hair even when dampened with lotion to conduct the current from the tweezers all the way down to the papilla, ensuring its destruction. Some therapists believe that the tweezer method, however, is excellent for blondes and Eastern or oriental women, who have very small follicles and very sparse and fine surplus hair. Electrolysis is an ideal if costly method of treatment for destroying facial hairs and for small areas of hair or areas of isolated hair growth, such as around the nipples, on a wart, and just to tidy up the slightly uneven, messy bikini line or bra line. Otherwise for women, particularly during the summer months or prior to a holiday, waxing is sufficient to ensure rapid, comfortable and relatively cheap, temporary hair removal. Effective waxing keeps the areas relatively hair-free for four to six weeks. Hairs grow back finer, especially after two to three sessions. It is important to remember though that some stubble growth of hair is needed for the wax to adhere firmly. Home do-it-yourself kits consist of prewaxed strips that you press on to the skin and then rip off, removing the hairs with it. This can also prove simple and effective. Hair removal creams based on chemicals such as calcium thioglyconate which dissolve the protein which makes up the hair, also give a smooth and silky finish and may be used on any part of the body including the upper lip, provided a patch test is first done to rule out risk of allergy or sensitivity. Wet or dry electric shaving can be used for underarms and legs but is not particularly suitable for the body and certainly not for the face. A point to remember: shaving does *not* stimulate or coarsen regrowth, but because hairs are sliced off bluntly in a straight line they re-emerge *feeling* coarser and more stubbly.

Pigmentary Problems

Chloasma

Those dark muddy brown patches of facial hyper-pigmentation which deepen in the sun, can prove a niggly and persistent problem for women who are pregnant or on the Pill. It is thought that in both cases increased levels of oestrogen stimulate melanocyte production and causes irregular blotchy areas, a result of photo-sensitivity. Although the patches, which generally appear on the upper lip, forehead, and around the eyes and crest of the cheek, do fade, they tend usually to become noticeably darker than the normal skin tone during exposure to sunlight. Applying a total sunblock will prevent further darkening, and in some cases a bleaching cream may successfully fade or eliminate the patches altogether. Commercial products like Fadeout and Esoterica contain very low amounts of hydroquinone bleaching agent — a mere 2 per cent — which may not be sufficient to have much impact on pigment. If the condition is severe, a doctor will prescribe a cream containing a higher percentage of hydroquinone or also other chemicals such as salicyclic acid to boost the bleaching process. The cream must be applied over a two to three-month period, twice a day on clean skin, and during this time a sunblock must be applied at all times before going into the sun. Bleaching agents are also known skin irritants and may unduly sensitise the skin causing redness and itching. An increasing number of dermatologists and plastic surgeons are using carbon dioxide liquid 'slush' to freeze off hyper-pigmented patches as well as other sundry blemishes and signs of sun damage and ageing. Though not technically chloasma, dark brown streaks and blotches can also appear on the body as a result of using a product, especially a perfume or cologne containing extract of bergamot, a known photo-sensitiser, and then going out into the sun.

Vitiligo

A much more distressing, unsightly and non-responsive condition is patches of depigmented skin which can affect any part of the face and body. Thought to be an auto-immune disorder which alters the body's normal production of the melanocyte-stimulating hormone, doctors still haven't fathomed out exactly how or why it occurs, although many believe it is triggered by stress and shock. Small patches of spots, especially those on the face, can often be realistically disguised with camouflage make-up, but larger areas of depigmentation may be treated by painting the white patches with a psoralen — a substance that makes the skin photo-sensitive — and then applying long-wave UVA 'black' light to stimulate the production of melanocytes. Unfortunately PUVA treatment, as it is called, only works in about 20 per cent of cases, usually proving only partially successful and giving the white patches a mottled appearance, and because as many as a hundred or more treatments may be needed before any improvement is seen, doctors are rightly concerned about the risk of skin cancer due to excessive UVA light exposure. Exposure to ordinary strong sunlight should also be avoided by anyone suffering from vitiligo, because far from evening out the condition, burning of the white areas and deepening of the normal surrounding skin will only compound the existing unevenness.

Pityriasis Versicolor (tinea versicolor)

This is the most innocuous, easily curable of all pigmentary disorders because it is caused by a fungus and as such has nothing to do with the body's production of melanin. Very common in hot, humid, tropical climates — about 80 per cent of all cases of pityriasis versicolor are found in the tropics — where fungi are prone to flourish, pityriasis may well appear like mild vitiligo, consisting of lots of smallish white or reddy-pink patches depending on basic skin tone usually covering the back, neck, chest or shoulders. The cause of the problem is a liophilic yeast which produces a toxin that kills off some of the skin's pigment cells allowing them to scale off. Pityriasis (also known as tinea versicolor) can be instantly diagnosed by a specialist and cured within three weeks with the use of an anti-fungal ointment such as Canestan or an anti-fungal shampoo used as a body disinfectant wash.

Fungal Infections

It may not be something we are immediately aware of but the healthy skin surface is covered with zillions upon zillions of microscopic plant organisms, which in normal conditions exist perfectly harmoniously and harmlessly, constantly maintaining the ecological balance of the skin, strengthening its anti-bacterial defences, and maintaining its pH levels. While these bacteria are vital to the maintenance of healthy skin, a lowering of the body's immune system, warm, moist environments, or direct internal or external infection can weaken this protective barrier, encouraging 'foreign' fungal infections to develop and thrive on the skin, giving rise to a broad spectrum of superficial skin infections. People who are immuno-suppressed (with a severely weakened immune system) such as those on cancer chemotherapy, radio-therapy, transplant patients, people suffering from AIDS (Acquired Immune Deficiency Syndrome), or people taking cortisone therapy are particularly liable to develop both super-ficial as well as systemic fungal infections because of the inability of the body's white cells to ward off the invading microbes. Their habits and habitats have fascinated microbiologists for decades and luckily, in recent years, there has been a welcome break-through in the treatment and control of a wide range of previously resistant fungal disorders. Scientists have developed new, fast-acting and effective anti-fungal treatments that can cure these infections with virtually 100 per cent success. The commonest skin fungus is tinea or ringworm, an umbrella-term used to describe a number of lesions but in particular raised red rings, sometimes of scaly patches covered in pustules, which appear on the body especially around the groin, the scalp, and the nail bed. The scaly patches are usually characterised by an inflamed edge and usually caught from animals, other infected humans or wet floors, for instance in communal changing rooms, swimming baths, etc, which are a breeding ground for such fungal infections. Probably the most familiar manifestation of ringworm is athlete's foot, which causes the familiar sogginess, scaling and cracking of skin between the toes. Highly inflamma-tory, itchy and contagious, ringworm seems to be more common in tropical countries and in people with asthma and hay fever, possibly due to a 'kink' in the body's immune system. Ringworm is easily curable with a short course of Nizoral tablets or long-term therapy with Griseofluvin, or a topical cream such as Tolnath, to destroy the fungus. Athlete's foot can usually be cleared up quite simply by regular washing and careful drying of the feet and toes and by the use of an anti-fungal powder or ointment to heal cracked skin and kill off the fungus. Anyone prone to foot infections should assiduously avoid skin contact with the floors of communal changing rooms, using other people's towels, socks, shoes, and walking barefoot in the gym and exercise studios.

Only too distressingly familiar to an overwhelming majority of women is the curdish discharge and general itch and embarrass-ment associated with thrush or candida, which is caused by a yeast-like fungus normally endemic in the gut and sometimes in the vagina. Vaginal thrush can and does flare up for any number of reasons, since the moist, warm, dark confines make this an ideal proliferation ground for fungal infection. Since the itching, soreness and discharge can signal any number of genital, urinary or sexually-transmitted diseases, symptoms must be diagnosed by a specialist, either privately or at a clinic, so that correct treatment can be prescribed. Taking the Pill, wearing tight nylon pants, tights, jeans, or taking antibiotics, is known to encourage thrush by altering the fine acid-alkaline ecological balance of the vagina. All these factors have contributed, say dermatologists, to its rise into almost epidemic proportions. Wearing an intra-uterine device or using a diaphram can also trigger thrush in some women, as can stress, hot humid weather, having diabetes, or being pregnant. Treatment is, however, fast, simple and in the majority of cases totally effective these days, although some women mysteriously seem more prone to chronic, intermittent or recurrent thrush than others. Most commonly prescribed are Nystatin or Nizarol tablets to destroy every vestige of thrush in the gut, usually used in combination with a clotrimazole-based anti-fungal vaginal pessary (Canestan) and/or cream. The simp-lest, fastest and least messy treatment for women with acute isolated attacks of thrush is the newest one: a tablet (Travogyn or Canestan tablets) inserted in the vagina at night which goes on working over a three-day period and can be safely taken by pregnant women — pregnant women are particularly prone to developing thrush. Men whose sexual partners are prone to thrush may sometimes develop the condition on their penis — symptoms consist of slight redness and the formation of small spots which can easily be treated and cured by applying an anti-fungal cream.

Thrush of the mouth is relatively common in babies, whose immune system is not yet fully developed, while in adults it can be caused through wearing ill-fitting dentures which allow saliva to permeate through the sides of the mouth. Thrush of the nails can affect women, especially those who spend a lot of time working with their hands in water, when the protective cuticle of the nail eventually wears off, opening up a gap between the nail bed and the nail plate and causing the yeast infection to imbed itself in and around the nail. Flesh around the nail then becomes raw, tender and cracked, while the nail itself can be riddled with dents and ugly grooves, becoming more and more porous as the combined effects of infection, detergents and water eat away at the nail surface, causing it to crumble away. Use of cotton-lined PVC gloves — rubber tends to encourage allergic reactions — is a must during all wet work and the hands should not be allowed to become hot and clammy. Nails and cuticles should be treated with an anti-fungal ointment every time the hands are washed. Remember, too, that thrush of the nails can also easily be passed on through contact to the genital area — yours and/or his — so your doctor will probably want to keep a close check on any skin irritation, itchiness or vaginal discharge that occurs while the patient is suffering from a nail infection. Men may be victims of sexually-transmitted cross-infection if their wives or sexual partners have thrush of the vagina, mouth or nails, and this usually shows up as a rash sometimes accompanied by small red spots or scaliness, which can easily be cured by the use of an anti-fungal cream. Any discharge, rash, swelling, soreness or unexpected lesions in the genital area in either men or women should be reported at once, either to a dermatologist or to the clinic for sexually-transmitted diseases at one of the large hospitals. Consulting a specialist or hospital clinic, rather than your local GP, greatly increases your chances of getting a fast and totally accurate diagnosis and correct treatment, since the experts are used to diagnosing and treating a very wide variety of major and minor genito-urinary-cum-skin problems, and they will probably be able to advise you promptly on the precise nature of the problem, thanks to a hawk-like trained eye and up-to-date sophisticated laboratory equipment.

Psoriasis

Although it has been estimated that 2 per cent of the population suffer from psoriasis, to sufferers and doctors it remains the biggest, most distressing dermatological riddle left to be solved. Not nearly as obvious or as uncomfortable as eczema since it doesn't itch and usually only affects the body and not the face, psoriasis usually appears on specific areas of the body — often those with less underlying flesh — such as the elbows, lower back, shoulders, knuckles, knees, and thighs, while 50 per cent of sufferers find the condition spreads to the scalp. Characterised by dull red plaques of any size, often round or oval in shape and covered in silvery scales which are rough to the touch, the spots can be very small and grow both in size and number, and they seem governed by an erratic, idiosyncratic time clock, sometimes flaring up and multiplying for a period and then fading for prolonged periods, settling into a stable pattern and remaining mild and unremitting for years on end, with unexpected remission when least expected. It is certainly the quirkiest of disorders and thus one of the most infuriating. In some rare cases the psoriasis takes on a yellowy, spotty rather than plaque-like appearance, especially on the hands and feet (pustular psoriasis), and it may also sometimes only affect the fingernails and toenails, discolouring, denting and pitting the nail surface and causing it to separate from the nail bed. The disorder can strike at any age but flares up prominently in the teens and twenties or in the fifties and sixties. Doctors believe the tendency to develop psoriasis is inherited; if one or both of your parents suffer from it, then you are more likely to be a sufferer. Statistics suggest that slightly more men than women tend to develop the complaint, but why it occurs no one knows, although according to Professor Ronald Marks of Cardiff University Medical Centre, no single skin disease is at present being more thoroughly researched since it is especially challenging, spilling over from the realms of dermatology into biochemistry, cellular biology and immunology. Like acne and eczema, full understanding of the nature of psoriasis can result only from the wide-angle not the narrow-lens approach of the skin specialists. Clues offered up by research in all these diverse fields suggest so far that psoriasis may well be an auto-immune disease whereby the body's immune defence system begins attacking not just foreign substances but also the body's own constituents, and is linked possibly to a defect in the white blood cells which invade scaly plaques in a specific and over-active way. There is some research to suggest that psoriasis sufferers share certain genetic traits on a cellular level with people who develop arthritis and other diseases. The most widespread theory to date, backed up by such sophisticated techniques for studying cells as scanning electron microscophy and 'freeze fracture', is that the walls of skin cells of those people suffering from psoriasis appear to have an in-built defect which makes the cells in psoriasis plaques join together abnormally — a significant factor, say dermatologists, since cell formation in any part of the body largely determines how body tissue grows and behaves. In fact cell kinetics — the study of the quantitive and qualititive changes in cell movement — is developing into a fascinating branch of dermatology and one which doctors believe will yield tremendously valuable information about the precise nature of a broad spectrum of disorders.

One thing is certain, although it could be a direct cause or an effect of the actual disorder, is that psoriasis is characterised by a very rapid cell turnover within the epidermis which accounts for the flaking and scaliness. Basal skin cells which normally take twenty-one to twenty-eight days to reach the skin's surface, may only take as little as four days to renew themselves. What is more, these cells have a tendency to clump and stick together more readily than in healthy skin. Abnormal expansion of the surface blood vessels and increased blood flow account for the redness of the condition. Psoriasis carries more aesthetic drawbacks than actual discomfort. About one in twenty sufferers may experience some form of related arthritis (conversely, one in twenty arthritis sufferers have psoriasis), which is known as psoriatic arthropathy and attacks mainly the joints at the ends of the fingers, causing swelling and pain. The jaw and joints in the lower back can also sometimes be affected. People with psoriasis may also experience localised forms of rheumatoid arthritis of the middle joint of the fingers and sometimes the wrists and ankles, which can flare up and disappear automatically. As with all skin disorders the psychological impact can prove a lot more undermining and devastating than the physiological disfigurement, causing, especially in young people, extreme embarrassment, lack of self-confidence, sexual inhibition and general depression. A lot of this certainly has to do with the ignorance and misconceptions that shroud the condition and make society in general still liable to recoil from, or stigmatise, anyone with noticeable skin lesions, under the misapprehension that they are infectious, represent lack of hygiene, or signify some dreaded internal disease. So although as yet there exists no known cure for psoriasis, it is vital to consult a skin specialist for treatment to improve, minimise, or at least control the condition, if not make it disappear altogether.

What Science has to Offer

Though often very effective, the creams and ointments used to treat psoriasis are notoriously messy and foul smelling, which is undoubtedly one of the reasons for the significant drop-out rate of users, who rate the therapy as worse than the condition. The two principle substances used are tar and dithranrol. Tar treatment, using a thick, black, oily, smelly ointment, sometimes blended with a salicylic acid to relieve scaliness, may be applied at home or as a daily part of a two-to-three-week hospital regime, and used in combination with ultraviolet light to speed healing. Staining of the clothes and bed linen can be prevented by using bandages over certain parts of the body. Dithranrol is a synthetic derivative of a substance called chrysarobin which occurs naturally in a number of plants. It is cytotoxic (poison cells) and very effective but highly potent, and it also stains clothes and bed linen permanently a dark brownish purple. Although it may irritate some skins, it works by dampening down accelerated cell turnover and improving surface scaliness. Dithranrol can be prescribed in varying strengths to suit the individual and may be used at home or, as with tar, as part of an intensive hospital-based therapy involving daily treatment and possible UV radiation as an adjunct.

Corticosteroid creams and ointments offer by comparison a seductively easy alternative. Bland, non-messy and easy to use they can greatly improve the condition, but are in essence suppressive, not healing, so that when therapy is stopped there is often a rebound action. Used extensively over the body and in very high doses of fifty or more grams a week, they can be absorbed into the system where they insidiously undermine the body's own manufacture of the hydro-cortisone needed to cope with stress and shock, increasing the risk of systemic infection and viruses. Even used in lower doses over shorter periods of time, corticosteroids tend to atrophy the skin, damaging the connective tissue and causing thinning, stretch marks, redness and increased susceptibility to fungal disorders and inflammation. Many dermatologists have become alarmed at the routine prescription, medical over-use and abuse of corticosteroid for a number of skin disorders, simply because the immediate improvement is often so spectacular and gratifying to both patient and doctor. Recently more and more doctors recognise that this is merely an easy way out in the short term, providing only temporary relief. What is more, as the disastrous side-effects of inappropriate corticosteroid therapy come to light, it seems the long-term repercussions even when merely cosmetic often far outweigh the immediate benefits.

Systemic Treatments

Compared to the hassle and mess of using standard topical psoriasis ointments the idea of just swallowing a pill to keep the condition under control appears a blissfully neat and uncomplicated answer, though this approach is somewhat drastic and not without its own particular risks. All internal psoriasis treatments are very powerful and thus fraught with potential side-effects, and it is therefore highly unlikely that a doctor will prescribe them for any other than the severest, most chronic forms of the disease. Methotrexate and razoxin are drugs often used to treat cancer including leukemia, Hodgkin's disease, and transplant patients. In the same way that it controls the division of malignant cells it also stops epidermal cells from dividing and reproducing at an unnaturally high rate. Therapy may last for six months to one or two years and possible side-effects include liver damage, digestive tract disorders, impaired bone-marrow function, and damage to the unborn fetus in pregnant women. Regular monitoring is therefore essential during its therapy. Tigason, a man-made vitamin-A compound or oral retenoid similar to 13-Cis retonic acid used to treat severe acne, and developed in the past ten years, is the latest shining hope in the treatment of very severe, unresponsive and pustular psoriasis — common psoriasis in contrast responds rather less well. Oral retinoids work particularly well in controlling the epithelial cells which constitute the 'lining' tissues of the body, as well as the faulty keratinisation such as the abnormally hyperactive cell activity associated with psoriasis. Tigason (medical name etretinate) has proved highly successful in reducing psoriasis although, as treatment is basically suppressive, the condition may reappear a certain period after treatment is stopped. It can only be administered under the strictest medical supervision, since side-effects include liver damage, increased levels of blood fats including cholesterol, and excessive dryness of the skin and membranes lining the mouth, nose, and eyes. Women taking oral retinoids must not get pregnant during therapy or for at least one year after, since the drug lingers in the system for a long time.

PUVA (Psoralen-UVA)
An acronym for psoralen UVA, PUVA (pronounced 'poo-va')

relies on the photo-sensitising properties of various plant extracts known as psoralens (oil of bergamot, parsley, dill, carrot, figs, are just a few) to intensify the healing properties of long-wave UV 'black' light. Effective as it undoubtedly has proved over the past few years in alleviating serious psoriasis, controversy hinges mainly on the risk of skin cancer, reports of which have so far emanated mainly from America. Because PUVA treatment is still relatively new, specialists say as yet it is too early to establish the extent of this risk, especially as it may take years after treatment for tumours to crop up. Because of these inherent drawbacks, treatment is only given to people over eighteen, although many doctors refuse to treat anyone with fair skin who is statistically more at risk of developing skin cancer. Therapy consists of swallowing a psoralen in pill form and one hour later exposing the affected areas to a UV light machine, rather like a solarium or sun lamp. Goggles are essential to prevent damage to the eyes. Nausea, vomiting, itching and burning of skin can be a problem in a minority of patients. PUVA therapy can only be given in hospitals or on an out-patient basis, and initial treatment may take three or four weeks or more depending on individual response to it. That ordinary sunlight appears to have a marked beneficial effect on psoriasis is a long, well-established fact. People who spend the summer months out of doors and take holidays in warm, sunny climates, often find the raw scaly patches diminish or even disappear altogether, only to proliferate and become more prominent as colder weather sets in. Why exactly UV rays should exert such a healing effect remains largely a mystery, although many doctors believe that it is the increased periods of rest, leisure time and relaxation connected with summer holidays and good weather which possibly contribute on a more subtle level to the improvement of psoriasis. Which all goes to underline the importance of cultivating mental and physical harmony and wellbeing as an antidote to psoriasis.

Natural Remedies

Stress, shock, nervous tension, anxiety, depression, and tiredness, though not in themselves a direct cause of psoriasis (with the possible exception of a severe emotional shock such as bereavement, which some specialists believe could be a catalyst in triggering the condition), are undoubtedly responsible for exacerbating the disorder, in the same way that chronic conditions like migraine and digestive upsets, for example, all tend to flare up when a person is under extreme physical and psychological pressure. There are certainly countless reported cases of temporary and long-term remission or improvement in eczema, psoriasis and arthritis when sufferers learn to reduce the degree of stress and tension in their lives, or to control their responses to stress factors by such popular deep relaxation methods as biofeedback, meditation, hypnotherapy, and autogenic training. If you suspect a link between your outbreak of psoriasis and the amount of stress and tension in your life, you can offer not only your skin but your mental and physical well-being and future health patterns no finer protection against the corrosive effects of stress than by studying one of these popular, well-established methods of deep mind/body relaxation. Alarmed and disenchanted with the high risk of side-effects from both topical and systemic psoriasis treatments, many sufferers are turning to natural remedies such as homeopathy and acupuncture which are often reported as having a highly beneficial effect in alleviating or at least controlling psoriasis as well as eczema. Over the past couple of years the Alternative Health Centre in London has been conducting research into natural alternatives to chemical drug therapy, in particular a range of Scandinavian treatments containing only natural herbs, mineral salts and worm wood, and essential plant oils. These are proving successful not only in relieving the dryness, redness and flakiness of psoriasis on the scalp and body, but also the itching and irritation of eczema. Dr Carl Pfeiffer of the Brain Biocentre in Princeton, New Jersey, points out that as far back as 1969 it was established that people with psoriasis have a low level of zinc in the body, and need more than the daily minimum requirement of the mineral to help counteract the disease. Large doses of zinc taken in combination with small doses of sulphur — best taken in the form of eggs — were used as far back as the nineteenth century to treat many skin disorders, and can not only sometimes provide relief from psoriasis but also from related arthritic complaints. Pyridoxine (vitamin B6) and riboflavin (B2) deficiency also seems to be a feature of psoriasis, and some studies show that when taken as an oral supplement both vitamins seem to improve the plaques and scaliness of psoriasis and the dryness and scaling of eczema. Certainly taking extra vitamins is not harmful — especially when compared to the side-effects of powerful cytotoxic drugs — and is worth trying over a period of time either as an initial therapy or if and when all orthodox treatment has failed.

Herpes

As the incidence of herpes assumes, in countries such as America, epidemic proportions, it has become the spectre of the 1980s and scourge of the sexually active — though by no means confined merely to the sexually promiscuous. Herpes is the blanket label given to a group of viruses which include the varicella-zoster virus responsible for chicken-pox in children and shingles in adults, and infectious mononucleuosis as well as the common and more emotive recurrent fever blisters or cold sores which affect the lips (herpes simplex 1) and genital infection (herpes genitalis 2). Despite massive scaremongering and sensationalist publicity over the present so-called epidemic of herpes 2 in particular, there still exists a tremendous muddle in many people's minds as to the exact nature of herpes and the finer points that differentiate the genital variety from the relatively mundane everyday cold sores. To begin with most specialists are agreed that while Hsv 1 and Hsv 2 can be separately identified, the symptoms are virtually identical and the virus which produces a cold sore on the lips can also cause genital sores — usually on the sides, near or just inside the vagina and within the buttock in women, or near the penis in males. While cold sores are more of an unsightly nuisance than anything else and are commonly triggered off by strong sunlight, colds, and menstruation, genital herpes on the other hand, especially in the case of a first attack, can, in the words of one doctor, be 'horrifically traumatic', accompanied by severe itching, excruciating pain and burning, caused by the blisters, and a general feeling of fatigue, nausea and fever, all of which can last from one to a few weeks until, under attack from the immune system, there is a spontaneous remission. Herpes of both varieties is *extremely* contagious and in fact can only be contracted through direct physical contact — most commonly through sexual intercourse, kissing, or any form of close physical contact whereby the active sores come into contact with another person's skin. When active, the herpes virus can sometimes penetrate even through the tiny invisible holes in a condom. Contrary to popular belief, you can pass herpes of the lips onto the genitals of another person during oral sex, while, conversely, having oral sex with someone suffering from genital sores will cause lip blisters. You can even cross-infect yourself — mouth to genitals or vice versa — simply by touching, perhaps unconsciously or in your sleep, the affected and non-affected areas. In very rare cases, a serious blinding eye disease called herpes keratitis may cripple certain people who have rubbed their eyes after touching either mouth or genital sores. Scrupulous hygiene, keeping blisters clear and dry and making sure not to touch them, avoiding skin contact, especially intercourse and kissing other people, is therefore absolutely vital in order to avoid transmitting the disease or aggravating the existing situation. There are various over-the-counter antiseptic soothing remedies, such as Anbesol, Herpid, and even calomine lotion, which will help to dry out and heal common cold sores, while Acyclovir (Zovirax ointment) is often prescribed by doctors to treat both types of outbreak. The reason why herpes 1 and 2 is such a vicious and scary infection is that to date it is incurable. Once a person has suffered an attack the virus remains with them for life, ever tenacious and ready to strike at any time. This is because once the blisters are treated or disappear the virus spontaneously takes refuge deep within the sacral ganglia — clusters of nerve cells situated near the spinal cord — where it lies dormant, safe from further attack by the body's immune system and ready to strike and cause a fresh outbreak at any time, be it every few weeks, months, or not for numerous decades. Some lucky people never experience a second outbreak and it seems that those who are run down or whose immune defences are depleted through illness, stress, shock or emotional trauma, AIDS, or those who are immuno-suppressed through powerful drug therapy, are more prone to recurrent attacks than someone with a strong constitution and a full quota of resources to fight off any virus or infection.

Future Hopes

Having thus staged a brilliant *coup d'etat* in order to ensure its lifelong survival, not for nothing is the herpes virus regarded as the ultimate parasite lurking now in a perfect hiding place ready to strike again given the appropriate catalyst. No wonder immunologists are facing one of the prime challenges of the decade in attempting to find an effective cure. So far the choices of effective treatment, let alone prevention or cure, are minimal. Clinical trials so far show that the anti-viral drug Zovirax when given internally for five days significantly reduces the pain and itching of genital herpes, accelerating the healing process by about 50 per cent. However the drug does not prevent the virus from becoming latent and therefore cannot protect against further outbreaks. Hopes are high in some medical circles that eventually everyone could be immunised against herpes as in the case of polio, German measles, etc. At the University of Birmingham, Dr Gordon Skinner is currently conducting a very encouraging three-year clinical trial into an anti-herpes vaccine based on preliminary studies which have shown that vaccination not only modifies the course of the disease in sufferers but also appears to protect over 90 per cent of the partners of known herpes sufferers. Better still, 75 per cent of patients who had experienced one attack were protected from further outbreaks by a series of injections of the vaccine. Encouraging though these results are, doctors remain cautiously optimistic and it will be some years before vaccination against herpes becomes routine treatment.

There is, however, some encouraging evidence that certain natural remedies may help to alleviate the worst symptoms of herpes and even damp down any recurrent attacks. In particular, naturopaths and homeopaths are enthusiastic about an amino acid called L-lysine, found in large quantities of foods such as potatoes, dairy produce, and brewer's yeast, and available in tablet form as a nutritional supplement. The beneficial effects of L-lysine in herpes sufferers were first discovered accidentally by Dr Chris Kagen in the Viral Laboratory at the Cedars of Lebanon Hospital in Los Angeles, when he noticed that another essential amino acid, L-arginine, was needed to enhance the growth of lab cultures of herpes viruses, while adding L-lysine had the opposite effect of actually retarding its growth. Theorising that L-lysine might well have a similar inhibiting effect on herpes in humans, he selected forty-five herpes patients and gave them between 300–1200 mg of L-lysine daily, suppressing symptoms in all except two cases. Better still, L-lysine in this study at least appeared to work therapeutically as well as prophylactically — monitoring some of these patients for up to three years later, Dr

Kagen's team noted that they suffered no recurrence of the disease. What is more, L-lysine is non-toxic and so has no adverse side-effects; it seems to get to work remarkably quickly, healing the blisters and removing the pain. However, L-lysine therapy does appear to be, like all other treatments, primarily suppressive, and so it must be ongoing — when patients stopped taking the amino acid their symptoms returned in one to four weeks. Researchers in this field have hypothesised that herpes sufferers may either eat insufficient L-lysine rich foods or else have an inherent inability to digest L-lysine properly from the food, or are quite simply unable to absorb the substance properly. In addition to L-lysine, the 'natural' approach to controlling herpes includes substances such as vitamin C, evening primrose oil — which has been found to improve chronic atopic eczema in children — zinc and vitamin E, all nutrients recognised for their ability to sooth and heal skin lesions. Women of child-bearing age suffering recurrent outbreaks of genital herpes, especially within the vagina, should undergo regular cervical 'pap' smear tests because they are potentially at a very high risk, since female genital herpes has been associated with a five to eight times increased incidence of cervical cancer, and as many as 50 per cent of babies born to women affected with herpes may suffer permanent brain damage or death. So concerned are doctors about this that they recommend all pregnant women with a history of herpes to undergo regular culture tests in the final trimester of their pregnancy, so that a caesarian delivery can be arranged if there is any sign of an outbreak of herpes around the time of the birth.

CHAPTER 9
Skin and the Environment

The miracle of human skin lies in its duality: surface delicacy belying life-long indestructibility, the ultimate multi-purpose consumer durable. A magnificent example of man's genetic adaptation to the environment, its nude smoothness, network of sweat glands, surface capillaries, increased layers of fat and outer keratin 'coating' all illustrate man's evolutionary emergence from dense jungle and forests to the open plains, the migration from warm sunny hemispheres to the colder, more hostile north. Skin is tough and resilient. And it has to be. The elemental wear and tear, the barrage of external stimuli and environmental insults to which human skin is constantly subjected and usually withstands often with minimal signs of distress, show how much we take this resilience for granted. But individual skin 'temperament' must inevitably dictate how many liberties we can take with our skin before it rebels against further punishment. The in-built ability of healthy skin to adjust itself according to changes in its environment does have certain limits, and it may develop a multiplicity of major and minor alarm signals which denote that it is either out of rhythm with itself or in discord with its environment. Dryness, flaking, chapped and cracked lips are the obvious and inevitable outcome of two very modern luxuries or everyday necessities, depending on which way you look at them: central heating and air conditioning. While the physical comfort that both these systems have brought to people whose lives would normally be abject misery in extreme weather conditions cannot be denied, nor can the fact that hot or cold, a dry atmosphere is a killer to skin. Air that lacks sufficient moisture wreaks havoc with the epidermis and epithelial tissues — the mucus membrane lining the nose, eyes and lips. A tight papery skin, and the formation of fine surface lines, are a particularly common complaint of anyone, particularly older people with normal or dry skin, while hot indoor atmospheres can also perversely stimulate the sebaceous glands to overreact in people with greasy, spotty, problem skins, giving a coarse pored, shiny complexion. Such symptoms are usually only temporary, but can be avoided by wearing a moisturiser, regular cleansing and freshening of the skin, constantly keeping a check on the level of temperature, opening windows, and installing humidifying units or placing bowls of water in the room to raise the moisture levels of the air. The drier the atmosphere the faster the water will evaporate, a sure sign that the skin's moisture reserves are in danger of depletion.

During the winter, humidity in centrally-heated buildings can fall to as low as 10 per cent, and even plummet right down to 0.2 per cent, which is about equivalent to the Sahara Desert at midday! Sleeping in an overheated room at night is a common cause not only of sinus congestion, but of fluid retention in the facial tissues, which accounts for the puffy complexion and baggy eyes many people suffer from when they get up, even after having enjoyed a good night's sleep. Keep the bedroom atmosphere as cool and moist as possible the year round to keep the skin from drying out or becoming puffy. Strong, ice-cold winter winds whipping against the skin are another seasonal hazard — greatly intensified on winter sports holidays in the Alps — that dry out and etch fine lines into the complexion. A rich emollient cream — perhaps a more heavy-duty formula than you might wear during warmer weather — will help guard the skin against chapping, flaking, redness, lines and dehydration. This is the time when a man's complexion can become raw, chapped and more irritated than usual by the combined assault of shaving and aggressive weather conditions, and the use of a moisturising cream or lotion and an embargo on harsh alcohol-based after-shave lotions can minimise discomfort, tightness and irritation as well as reduce the risk of premature ageing.

The discomfort often suffered during and after long-distance flights is largely caused through bodily dehydration, a direct result of spending prolonged periods in a pressurised atmosphere. Skin quickly becomes dry, tight, and covered in fine superficial lines, while the tissues beneath can become congested and swell up quite dramatically. Many of these temporary side-effects can be counteracted or alleviated by drinking plenty of water and fruit juices during and after the flight to replenish body fluids and by constantly applying rich facial moisturiser and hand and body lotion. Avoid alcohol, which dehydrates the body further, and caffeine-based drinks like tea, coffee and coca-cola, which work similarly by acting as a diuretic.

Sunshine — A Burning Issue

Harsh winds, however, lack of humidity, and positive ions are nothing compared to what scientists now know to be the most formidable environmental foe of all: natural sunlight. Its role as the skin's arch enemy number one is all the more devastating since its effects are misguidedly self-inflicted in the name of fashion and the erroneous assumption that because we do look healthier and sexier with a tan, it follows that a tan is synonymous with good health. As it now turns out, there is ever new and disturbing evidence that indeed the opposite may be true. If we could turn our skin inside out and examine the insults and injuries perpetrated in the name of fashion and glamour, doctors believe suntanning would soon be remembered merely as a quaint, self defeating and destructive ritual. Sunbathing of course is not a uniquely twentieth-century pastime. It goes back to classical Greek times. The historian Herodotus, writing around the time of 480 B.C., said 'exposure to the sun is eminently necessary to those who are in need of building themselves and putting on weight'. A prescient observation of the sun's role in vitamin-D synthesis and its ability to make us feel relaxed. Undeniably sexy, synonymous, though often wrongly, with spanking good health, a golden suntan is universally regarded nowadays as nature's most stunning cosmetic, but it may also turn out to be her deadliest. Yet such is the cachet attached to sporting bronze skin during the summer months or on a visit to hot, sunny countries, that most people continue to ignore dermatologists' warnings about the very grave potential hazards of sun worship. Doctors are now unanimously agreed that there is no vestige of doubt that over-exposure to strong ultraviolet light is the single and most lethal contributory factor to premature skin ageing and skin cancer in the world today. While the Elizabethans poisoned their skins with arsenic and lead to achieve a fashionable pallor, we in turn are perhaps well on our way to doing the same by cultivating brown skin.

Not that many people, especially those who tan deeply and easily and thus complacently without undue discomfort, are often aware of it. Tan now, pay later — perhaps not until ten, fifteen or twenty years' time — is the message; for sun damage begins slowly and insidiously, deep within the basal cell layers and deeper still within the dermis, to manifest itself only years later in the form of blotchy, dehydrated, thinning, wrinkled and prematurely lined, discoloured skin. Repeated over-exposure to strong sunlight, a formidable harbinger of free radicals incidentally, is the most common cause of degenerative changes in the tissues — what dermatologists call solar elastosis — and cross-linkage of the skin's collagen and elastin fibres with all that this implies in terms of surface ageing. For the skin is pre-programmed to overreact automatically in self-defence to the effects of sunlight. The results of this hyperactivity, according to Dr Albert Kligman, is that the sun-damaged skin has *too much* of everything — too much thickened epidermal tissue, too many overworked sebaceous glands and sweat glands, over-dilated capillaries, too many wrinkles, open pores and freckles, over-pigmentation, and brown 'age' spots. What is less known is that these unsightly degenerative changes actually begin very early in life if a person exposes their skin to the sun, even during childhood. Few doctors mince their words about this, and it is a chastening thought that most of the visible effects of ageing skin that emerge when a man or woman reaches their late thirties or forties represents the cumulative net result of sun damage incurred back in their teenage years. The correlation between the very steep and rapid increase in skin cancer worldwide and increased exposure to sun because of emigration to countries in the southern hemisphere, longer periods of leisure time spent outdoors, and holidays in hot sunny countries, is something that worries doctors a lot more.

As early as 1896 Dr Paul G. Unna, a German dermatologist, first suspected a link between sunlight and skin cancer — a suspicion now all too accurately confirmed. In 1900 cancer was responsible for one out of twenty-five deaths; today it is one in six, and one out of every four cancers today is a skin cancer. In America, where vast sections of the population are exposed to strong sunlight for a large percentage of the year, half a million new cases of skin cancer are reported each year, while the high percentage of skin cancer in countries such as South Africa, Australia, New Zealand, and the southern parts of the USA, has long been attributed to the effects of prolonged intensive ultraviolet radiation on people originally of Celtic origin with fair skin and hair, and blue/green/grey eyes. Doctors are increasingly concerned about those of us who live in temperate, relatively unsunny climes such as England, and subject our skins increasingly to a two or three-week intensive 'blast' of very strong sunlight. A recent study carried out by dermatologists at the University of Glasgow suggests that the most serious skin cancer, malignant melanoma, is caused by sudden exposure to intense sunlight, as when someone who normally lives in a cool, overcast environment most of the year spends a fortnight or three weeks bombarded by fierce and strong sunlight. Cases of malignant melanoma now represent 2 per cent of all cancers and 1 per cent of all cancer deaths and have more than doubled in the last ten years — with more cases reported after 'record' hot, sunny British summers (i.e. '76) — a trend that goes a certain way to substantiate the theory that increased leisure time, holidays in the tropics or the Mediterranean and other hot countries may be responsible for the increase in skin cancer.

The long and short of it

In order to understand not only the nature of tanning but also its concomitant dangers, it helps to visualise the changes that occur when we expose our skin to the sun. Sunlight hits the earth in varying frequencies or wavelengths that are measured in Nanometers. These range from infra-red heat (about 800 Nanometers) to ultraviolet or visible light of three distinct types.

UV-C rays (290 Nanometers) are blocked off from the earth's surface by its protective ozone layer. These are bacteriocidal and destroy germs, and they are used in laboratories for sterilisation procedures.

UV-B rays (290/320 Nanometers) are almost totally responsible for sunburn. Ninety per cent of these short-wave rays are absorbed into the epidermis; 10 per cent penetrate deeply into the dermis to create permanent damage. UV-B is absorbed by window-glass.

UV-A rays (320/400 Nanometers) are responsible for the synthesis of vitamin D and were thought until recently to be harmless to the skin, since they don't burn but do eventually stimulate tan. Scientists, however, now believe that because these long-wave rays are absorbed by the deepest layers of the dermis, they are ultimately responsible for degenerative changes within the connective tissue, the collagen and elastin fibres, and the DNA of cells, causing slower, more long-term skin damage. UVA light has recently been harnessed in two ways, firstly in conjunction with psoralens, plant extracts which act as photo-sensitising agents in PUVA treatment for psoriasis (psoralens plus UV-A) and in solaria and sunbeds to produce tanning without risk of burning.

Paradoxically the quest for cleaner air may have a 'kickback' effect, according to some scientists, by potentiating the damaging effects of ultraviolet light. Reduced pollution, for example, obviously allows more pure sunlight to filter through into the atmosphere, so clean air may hold a greater threat to those people already exposed to strong sunlight. Recently there has also been concern that propellents in aerosols and supersonic flights could theoretically destroy this ozone layer, which in turn could lead to future generations suffering radiation damage.

The skin's major defence against burning is its capacity to synthesise melanin to a degree that varies greatly from person to person and is genetically programmed. Those most prone to burning are people with blue, grey, or green eyes, fair or red hair, and fair or freckled skin which has a low malanin quota and burns easily. Dark coloured and black skinned people have an in-built, ready-made pigmentary 'armour' that serves as a first line of defence against burning and skin damage. Melanogenesis — commonly known as tanning — is stimulated by UV-B and UV-A radiation as an automatic self-protective mechanism against burning. As sunlight is absorbed by the skin, tyrosinase, an enzyme present in the melanocytes (pigment cells) of the basal layers, is activated, causing the transformation of tyrosin, a colourless amino-acid, into melanin, a colourful molecule which migrates upwards to the surface of the skin giving it its characteristic golden or bronze tan. The more melanin is produced, the darker the tan and the greater the amount of energy absorbed from the sun's rays, preventing radiation from damaging the epidermis. Unfortunately some people never produce enough melanin to provide sufficient UV protection, and because of the relatively slow nature of the tanning mechanism, most skins undergo a certain amount of irreparable and significant damage prior to and in the process of acquiring a tan. Therefore by the time you go brown — with the exception of those with very dark olive 'Mediterranean-type' skin who turn brown within one or two days — the damage is already done.

The most savage aspect of the sun's assault on skin is undoubtedly caused through burning, which even on a mild scale quickly damages the epidermis by (a) overheating and dehydrating the tissues, and (b) producing erythema, an inflammatory reaction which dilates and weakens the blood vessels, causing the tissues to swell and fill with fluid which later leads to the formation of blisters and peeling. A further self-defence process is triggered by accelerated cell renewal causing thickening of the epidermis which, like a tan, absorbs energy and prevents the sun's rays from reaching the dermis. It is this toughening up of the epidermis which, along with overheating of the tissues and dilation of the blood vessels, accounts for the lined, coarse texture of the skin after initial exposure to the sun — temporary effects that nevertheless accumulate over years of sun worship, leading to permanently dehydrated skin, broken dilated capillaries and premature lines, wrinkles, and loss of elasticity caused by a gradual weakening and breakdown of the skin's underlying supportive collagen and elastic fibres. The fairer your skin, the greater the fuel for the sun's rays and the more acute and long lasting the degree of havoc wrought on the skin through burning, over-exposure, and insufficient protection.

Bearing in mind this long litany of woes familiar to anyone who has ever been the victim of sunburn, it does seem incredible that year after year one can still observe the beaches and sun spots of the world littered with the pink-skinned peeling casualties of irresponsible, over-zealous sun worship. Ignorance and a short memory, as well as damaged skin, characterise the foolhardy sunbather. For what is often overlooked is that red today does not mean brown tomorrow, for the two processes are quite different; burning (erythema) is caused through dilation and damage of the blood vessels which sends blood coursing to the skin's surface causing it to go red; tanning is due to melanin synthesis, and the two processes are *not* mutually inter-dependent or even compatible.

Fail Safe

The visible, seemingly transient but certainly acute, short-term effects of burning, blisters, redness, peeling, and soreness are of course well established as the prime cause of surface damage. These acute short-term effects are further compounded by slower accumulated degenerative changes that take place deep within the dermis over a longer period of time — changes which in themselves have nothing to do with burning but which principally involve damage to the epidermis. Thanks to the pioneer research work carried out into the nature of skin ageing and the effects of ultraviolet light by leading dermatologists like Dr Albert Kligman, this insidious and subtle transmutation of healthy living tissue is, according to many scientists, probably caused not just by UV-B light but by those so called 'safe' and benevolent long-wave UV-A rays which dig far deeper into the dermis and wreak slow but cumulative changes that only show up years later. For a good example of what dermatologists are now talking about, one need only look at the leathery, lined, yellowy, coarse-grained complexions of middle-aged and elderly women who spend their days soaking up the sun in say Florida, or the teenagers and twenty-year-old Israelis who already sport crow's feet and deep nose to mouth lines, normal expression lines whose form and depth have been accelerated by the sun.

A lot of nonsense is often bandied around about 'safe' UV-A and 'unsafe' UV-B rays. But if UV-A light can cause the photochemical reactions inside cells that lead to tanning — most obvious to anyone who uses a sunbed for a few sessions of instant tanning — then it follows that it can also instigate other more harmful effects. Absorbed by the collagen and elastin protein that supports the connective tissue, UV-A light gradually weakens and breaks up strands of DNA, the genetic material within the cell nucleus. Although enzymes are constantly at work to excise damaged sections of DNA and rearrange the DNA strands into their proper sequence, repeated UV-A exposure can cause this repair system to break down, allowing the formation of chemical cross-links within the DNA that then cause the cell to replicate itself incorrectly. The result? Accelerated skin ageing, the formation of benign growths and skin tumours — solar keratoses — or worse, skin cancer. Skin cancer is UV's final insult. Incorrectly-repaired mutated cells can eventually proliferate and cause the formation of malignant growths, especially on exposed and vulnerable areas such as the lips, ears, forehead, and cheeks which the sun's rays hit hardest. Luckily skin cancer, being noticeable, can be detected in its early stages and treated successfully before it spreads to the rest of the body. Skin cancer usually stems from the basal cells, and the risk of developing cancer, like becoming prematurely-aged, is directly proportional to the amount of sun exposure and inversely proportional to the colour of a person's skin. The darker the skin the more sun it can take with less risk of cancer and ageing, the fairer the skin the greater the dangers. Location is another contributory factor: the incidence of skin cancer *per capita* doubles every two hundred miles nearer the equator and is rife, for instance, in countries like South Africa, Australia, and the southern states of America.

Early-warning signs of cancer may take the form of solar keratoses, crusty red wart-like lesions that appear on the face or backs of the hands and refuse to heal. Though premalignant, these must be removed promptly to eliminate any future risk of malignancy. Basal cell carcinoma, or rodent ulcers, consist of a malignant single spot with a round, shiny or pearly surface and a depressed central crater which slowly spreads and grows into the surrounding area, but does not spread to other parts of the body via the blood or lymph system (i.e. metastasise). Squamous cell carcinoma, which also forms on some exposed areas, can metastasise and appears as a rough, scaly, brown, red or beige spot with an irregular shape and a tendency to bleed. If it occurs near the mucus membranes — lips, ears, eyes, nose — it has a greater chance of spreading through the circulatory system. Most deadly of all is a malignant melanoma which stems usually from a pigmented mole and need be no larger than a halfpenny to kill. It has probably the worst prognosis of any cancer in the body, despite its advantage of being readily seen. Unfortunately most people, especially men, have a tendency to ignore skin growths or procrastinate in visiting a doctor when they develop a suspicious skin lesion, building up a time-lapse which can prove fatal. Malignant melanoma, however, *can also be cured* by surgery, like a rodent ulcer or squamous cell carcinoma, if it is caught in the very early stages before the tumour has taken hold too deeply and spread to other areas of the body to create life-threatening secondary cancers. Most disconcerting of all in respect of the known correlation between sun exposure and cancer is some recent evidence which suggests that UV radiation may not cause cancer merely by causing mutagenic skin changes, but also by immuno-suppression — undermining the proper function of the body's disease fighting surveillance and 'warrior' enzymes which, in turn, encourages the growth of cancer. Margaret Kripke of America's National Cancer Institute has demostrated that mice exposed to small doses of UV don't reject transplanted tumours as readily as they normally would, and tests carried out at Massachusetts General Hospital, Boston, and Sydney Hospital, Australia, suggest that UV alters the efficiency and function of the lymphocytes, the white blood cells involved in the immune reaction to foreign tissue. Inconclusive and fragmented as it is, such evidence might help to explain why malignant melanoma often appears on those areas of the body, for instance the buttocks, not normally exposed to the sun, although the victim has received prolonged intensive UV exposure elsewhere, and why people infected with the herpes simplex virus develop fever blisters after exposure to strong sunlight.

Sense and Sensibilities

In contrast to this gloomy scenario, dermatologists are quick to point out that we do not necessarily have to cover ourselves with veils or big hats, carry parasols or shun the outdoors in order to avoid premature ageing and/or skin cancer. Although eschewing sunlight and espousing shade is of course the finest guarantee of maintaining a youthful and healthy complexion well into middle age and beyond, scientific expertise has ensured that the sunscreen and sunblock preparations on the market today meet very high standards of efficiency, allowing people with even very pale and sensitive skins to go into the sun without the risk of burning and allowing others to develop a tan slowly over long periods of time with minimal risk of damage to their skin. Skin damage is therefore easier to prevent now than ever before in man's history. The degree of protection offered by today's sunscreens is in direct proportion to its in-built protection factor (PF), ranging usually from two or three, which offers minimal protection from burning, to eight or ten, ideal for someone who wants to tan slowly and safely over a longer period of time without any risk of burning, right up to a fifteen, eighteen, twenty-five or total sunblock, which gives maximum coverage ensuring that you will neither burn nor tan. Specialists such as Dr Albert Kligman involved in the study of ageing skin and the effects of UV light stress that *everyone*, regardless of their skin type and especially babies, young children and teenagers, who spend most amounts of time out of doors in strong sunlight, should wear a PF of fifteen to avoid the sort of cumulative, deep-down, long-term, degenerative changes of which most of us remain blissfully unaware and which only manifest themselves later in life. So strong is his conviction as to the very real long-term dangers of all varieties of UV-A radiation, that Dr Kligman advocates that even men, women and children who live in a temperate climate such as that of Great Britain should protect their skins with a high-factor sunscreen all the year round, even during a sunny day in winter. As he sees it, we should all seriously rethink our conditioned responses to sunlight, beginning with the realisation that in very hot climates, the damage of sunlight as born out by the latest research is not merely skin deep. Dividing sunlight up into 'good' and 'bad' rays is also a pointless exercise, since radiation from sunlight is polychromatic. 'You don't just get one slice of the UV spectrum, you get the whole package, including infra-red in the form of heat which is also very damaging to skin.'

Responding to such warnings in deadly earnest, many of the major cosmetic companies are now incorporating sunscreens into make-up and skin-care ranges, and even into eye make-up and lipsticks, while constantly refining and improving the texture of sunscreen products to suit all skin types, even those that are greasy, prone to spots and acne, or very allergy-prone and sensitive. So there is absolutely no reason for anyone to risk burning or damaging their skin nowadays. Recent improvements include alcohol-free, non-perfumed products to suit sensitive skins and water-resistant formulae that adhere better to the skin and are less likely to come off with perspiration or during swimming.

The Cover Story

For obvious reasons the best sunscreen products filter out all the burning UV-B rays and also a certain percentage of long-wave UV-A rays. The most reliable chemicals used as UV-B and UV-A sun-screening agents are PABA (para-amino benzoic acid), cinnoxate, padimate O, ethylhexyl methoxy cinnamate, or one of the benzophenone group of derivatives. These can cause irritation in certain people, though true allergic reaction is rare. Some people who are allergic to sulphonamides (a group of antibiotics), hair dyes and benzocaine and other anaesthetics are more likely to develop an allergy to the p-amino benzoate and its derivatives. The greatest protection of all — 100 per cent block of both UV-B and all UV-A rays — comes from total sun-blocking agents containing opaque chemicals such as zinc oxide and titanium dioxide, which deflect the sun's rays. These products are absolutely essential protection for anyone taking photo-sensitising drugs such as tranquillisers or antibiotics, or other topical medication that can render the skin photo-sensitive, anyone suffering a disorder that can cause photo-sensitivity or photo-allergy of the skin, and people suffering from acne rosacea, albinism, and any allergic reactions which occur in direct response to sunlight. Perhaps the whole messy business of rubbing on sunscreens throughout the day may one day, however, become a thing of the past, making life on holiday a lot easier. Doctors at Harvard Medical School are working on developing a sunscreen pill that would inactivate certain forms of oxygen that are generated by UV light and cause cell membrane damage and other degenerative changes linked to skin cancer. Animal experiments are encouraging and have shown that it is possible to block the burning process as well as prevent other chemical and biological reactions by using an oral sunscreen, but such a product will not be available for human beings in the foreseeable future.

However the best sunscreen or sunblock in the world can be rendered useless if it is used incorrectly. Protective creams and lotions should always be applied before going into the sun and liberally reapplied during the day, especially after swimming and water sports, and after you have been sweating a lot and have wiped the product off with a towel, tissue, etc. What is more, skin can get burnt under the most deceptive conditions. An overcast sky can allow up to 50 per cent of the sun's UV-A and UV-B rays through; whilst sitting under an umbrella or canopy, UV light can still be reflected up at you from light, bright surfaces, such as concrete, snow and sand; and you can get burnt at 9 or 10 a.m. if you go out say for a long walk on the beach or play tennis without protection. The vulnerability of skin varies with age and health; just because you have never been burnt does not mean you can't, especially if you find yourself in those conditions where sunlight can be at its most lethal — between 11 a.m. and 4 p.m. out at sea, where the breeze takes the heat out of the rays, in high altitudes where less atmospheric filtration allows more UV-A rays through, when your body is wet and so admits more UV-A rays, and of course on the beach and next to water, snow and reflective surfaces. Parents with babies, children and teenagers who are constantly on the go in and out of the water and rubbing their skins, should pay particular attention that a sunscreen is re-applied throughout the day, especially on those parts of the body that are regularly uncovered. There are certain danger zones which remain the same at any age, and it is easy to forget that unlike any other light, sunlight is not beamed at us like a searchlight but is diffuse and scattered, which accounts for those mystery blotches and burns where one part of the body 'just happened to catch the sun'. Danger zones include the neck — often caught at a sideways angle by the sun's rays — the eyelids, the area around the crest of the cheek and the eye-socket, where the reflection of the sun bounces off the frame of sunglasses, the tops, sides and lobes of the ears, the hands, the nape of neck, and the legs and feet. Lips unlike other skin do not contain melanin and burn more easily — the mouth is a prime site for skin cancer. Sunlight can also prove dangerous and permanently damaging to the eyes. Apart from cultivating crow's feet and wrinkles from squinting, UV radiation denatures proteins in the lens of the eye, causing a slow deposit of yellow pigment that, like melanin, protects the retina from damage. Excessive accumulation of this pigment, however, has been shown to cause cataracts, which is why it is worth investing in a good pair of sunglasses that absorb both UV-B and UV-A light. Most tinted lenses cut out UV-B perfectly well, but in reducing visible light they make the iris dilate and the pupil open to allow even more UV-A into the eye. Contrary to the claims of many beauty salon owners and beauty therapists, goggles, cotton wool pads or some form of protection *must always* be worn over the eyes when you are undergoing sun treatment in a solarium or on a sunbed. Even short-term exposure of the naked eye to the very strong form of UV-A light used on sunbeds carries a very small risk of eventual damage to the eye and even blindness.

Repair Work

But once those degenerative changes have taken hold of the skin and it begins to age visibly, doesn't the concept of sun protection become rather academic? Absolutely not, according to Dr Albert Kligman whose studies involving both animals and humans suggest that a certain amount of sun damage is actually reversible. His most recent research involves a group of retired and hospitalised or institutionalised elderly men who had worked out of doors most of their lives and had severely weathered, sun-damaged skin. Just after their retirement, Dr Kligman took biopsies of sun-induced facial tumours, blotches, and solar keratoses, and again seven to ten years later, a period these elderly men had spent almost exclusively indoors out of the sun. Dr Kligman observed that most of these tumours had regressed and that the structure and appearance of the skin had improved with increased collagen synthesis. Of course it isn't necessary to spend the rest of your days indoors in order to repair or prevent sun-damaged skin. In controlled experiments involving laboratory animals, Dr Kligman has proved that sunscreens prevent the elastosis caused by UV light on normal healthy skin, but if a sunscreen is applied to skin already suffering elastotic damage and the skin is then further subjected to UV radiation, the area of skin that has been protected by the sunscreen actually repairs and renews itself, forming healthy new collagen on top of the old diseased connective tissue. All this is surely encouraging news and a tremendous argument in favour of staying out of strong sunlight and/or wearing a high PF sunscreen, even if you have already incurred a fair amount of premature ageing in years gone by. In other words, says Dr Kligman, it is never to late to begin protecting your skin from the sun, and the improvement in your skin may turn out to be well worth the effort. For one thing, he stresses, taking precautions at *any age* can prevent the formation of skin cancer, since every day spent in the sun could prove more harmful and, as he puts it, 'insulting to the skin'.

Faking It

In the light of current suspicions about the comparative safety of UV-A rays, probably one of the most specious arguments put forward by beauticians is that acquiring tan on a sunbed, which emits UV-A light only, offers an altogether safer alternative to lying in the real sun. Dr Kligman, like most dermatologists today, is adamant that sunbeds, like sun, can cause eventual premature ageing and pose a potential risk of cancer on two counts: possible 'contamination' of UV-A rays with a small but significantly damaging percentage of UV-B rays, and the risk of long-term accumulated degenerative changes within the dermis from UV-A radiation.

The photo-chemical changes which occur in skin tissue under artificial UV-A light are analogous to those that occur in natural sunlight if you wear a sunscreen that blocks out all the UV-B, except that the bombardment of UV-A is many thousand times greater than anything experienced in even very strong sunlight — hence that much vaunted 'instant' tan which makes sunbeds such an attractive proposition, especially in Britain. Although it certainly is safer to acquire a tan under artificial intensive UV-A light rather than risk going through the burning process in real sunlight, the question of safety remains relative: the damaging effects of UV-B are well documented, but with new evidence regarding the supporting role of UV-A in skin ageing and cancer, probably *neither* method is advisable to those who value the long-term youth and health of their skin. What is more, sunbeds are a relatively recent invention and so, as when the contraceptive pill was first introduced, the possible ill-effects cannot possibly be quantified or ascertained probably until the present generation of young men and women who regularly use sunbeds has reached middle or old age. There are certainly constant reports of the risks of skin cancer to psoriasis patients taking PUVA therapy, which involves taking photo-sensitising drugs and exposing the skin to intensive 'black' UV-A light. As photobiologist Dr Anthony Young sees it, the risks many people run when they take a course of sunbed sessions is that so called 'pure' UV-A light may well be contaminated, however slightly, by a fraction UV-B wavelength, which raises the risk of skin damage considerably. Many sunbed manufacturers — not to mention the salon owners who operate them — are often quite ignorant of the exact nature of the UV light emitted by the beds because they in turn receive the strip bulbs direct from the lighting manufacturers. An artificially cultivated tan is, contrary to popular belief, not as protective when you go into the real sunlight as its natural counterpart, because skin thickening, the body's other defence against burning, doesn't occur on a sunbed. So while pre-tanning is of great cosmetic value, reducing the compulsion to stay out too long and fry the skin in the early stages of the holiday in an attempt to develop a healthy skintone, the need to protect the skin with a high PF sunscreen remains the same. Other forms of artificial tanning are by comparison to sunbeds harmless to the skin, although they are unlikely to give as realistic a tan as one would obtain from a sunbed.

There are creams and lotions which give the skin a tanned appearance within a few hours by staining the outer layers. These artificial tanning agents were first introduced in the late 1950s and are based on a harmless cold tar derivative dihydroxyacetone (DHA), which produces a yellow-brown shade by reacting with the keratin to form pigments called melanoidines. Pills such as Orobronze work from the inside out to tan skin brown and are based on beta-carotene, a pro-vitamin A derivative, and a substance called canthaxanthin, which 'tones down' yellow skin coloration. Carotenoids are a group of widely occurring vegetable and animal pigments responsible, for example, for giving fruit bright coloured peel as well as birds such as flamingoes their pink, red and orange plumage. Doctors believe that the carotenoid in artificial suntanners does not raise the body's vitamin-A levels — unlike other mammals, man lacks the conversion process to do so — and are therefore safe to use cosmetically. Widely used as colourants in the food industry, both chemicals are used medically to reduce the unpleasant skin symptoms suffered by people, for example, with porphyria, whose skins are abnormally sensitive to UV light, imposing troublesome restrictions on open air life and holidays. In France particularly, both substances have proved popular as artificial suntanners.

Although psoralen-based sunscreens such as the original Bergasol formula to help skin turn brown faster have recently been taken off the market because of concern over cancer risks, there is still tremendous controversy regarding the links between psoralens and skin cancer in man. Psoralens — agents which sensitise the skin to UV-A — are a group of naturally occurring substances in the plant world first used in Egypt over 2,000 years ago to aid tanning. Parsley, citrus extracts including oil of bergamot, dill, figs, carrots; turnips, and parsnips are just some of the well-known natural psoralens. The recent furore centres around the substance called 8 MOP (methoxypsoralen), a psoralen commonly used in PUVA, and a variant of this, 5 MOP, which used to be included in very small quantities in products such as Bergasol. As with so many laboratory studies, the crux of the issue lies in the difference between mice and men. Applied to hairless mice 8 and 5 MOP does induce skin cancer under UV radiation; but then the ubiquitous hairless mouse, the subject of endless research into the damaging effects of everything from hair dyes to saccharine, is renowned as a short-lived, extremely vulnerable species which develops cancer or responds adversely to all manner of substances. Further, the research is done with purified chemicals, not the extracts used in suntan oils, and the quantities of psoralen given to these animals is far in excess of the amounts used in PUVA, let alone in a sunscreen, where the amounts are fractional. Precise and honourably carried out it may be, but such statistical or epidemiological evidence is vastly misleading, especially when it makes sensational front page exposé news, often causing instant panic and unnecessary worry and anxiety for millions of consumers who are not given all the correct facts. As it stands today though, 5 MOP is regarded as a possible carcinogen; the Board of Trade states that there is so far insufficient evidence of the harmful effects of 5 MOP to merit an investigation into suntan oils containing psoralens, which makes a certain amount of sense when you consider that many perfumes, colognes, and after-shaves contain oil of bergamot, a prime source of psoralen, as indeed does Earl Grey Tea! At the time of writing, however, most of the manufacturers of sun-screens containing extracts of psoralen or 5 MOP have in fact withdrawn their products from the market or altered the formulae.

CHAPTER 10
The Inside Story

As a primary sensor reponsible for transmitting physical or psychic messages of the utmost subtlety and complexity, the skin has no equal. The frequencies through which skin 'broadcasts' on the state of the individual can vary, ranging from the lowest of signals encompassing shifts and modulations in colour, texture, and contour to others of an unmistakable high pitch — outbreaks of eczema, oedema, hives, and shingles, that flaunts itself vividly to the world at large. Like litmus paper which reacts to changes imposed both within and without its structure, skin tissue is capable of yielding a myriad clues about how different human beings eat, drink, sleep, and generally nurture or neglect themselves.

Despite the assertion of many diehard conservative doctors to the contrary, the skin on our face, scalp and body offers lifelong living evidence of the changes that can be wrought — for better or worse — upon its outer appearance from the inside. To many dermatologists or general practitioners, a clear, healthy attractive skin may simply be one unscathed by the trauma of some unsightly disease or affliction. But like good health — which is by no means the same as absence of illness — a good skin, one which is in optimal health, offers a reflection of the food we eat, the drugs, drinks and stimulants we take, the amount of stress, shock, joy or relaxation we experience. To those therapists practising natural health, preventive or 'holistic' medicine, for example acupuncturists, homeopaths, and naturopaths, mind and body with all their component parts function as one single, interacting, interdependent unit. Skin problems like any other symptom of ill health or malaise cannot therefore be treated or diagnosed in isolation from the rest of the body. According to the holistic credo, to treat surface problems alone is merely to suppress them temporarily, allowing the root cause, be it nutritional or psychological in origin, to perpetuate further symptoms *ad infinitum*. The difference between the way an orthodox medical doctor or dermatologist and a holistic healer looks at the skin is one of dimension and degree of detail — the wide-angle lens versus the narrow close up, the panoramic 3D picture set next to the 2×4 identikit. To the trained eye, the shifting minutiae of skin colouring, texture, tone, lines, temperature, and secretions speak volumes not only about a person's individual skin 'profile' but also about what goes on deep down inside its structure. For instance, while most of us are well aware that eating a healthy, well-balanced diet will keep us looking and feeling our best, there is increasing evidence to suggest that certain nutrients are directly implicated in maintaining, repairing and renewing healthy skin tissue and preventing the degenerative changes associated with ageing and neglect.

Nutrition

The most extreme example of a link between diet and skin occurs in those people suffering from atopic eczema which, according to an increasing number of specialists, seems to occur as a result of an abnormal reaction of the immune system to certain foods. Normally, after you eat a meal, protein is broken down by the digestive enzymes into its constituent amino acids, which are then absorbed into the system through the gut wall. However, entire protein molecules may remain unprocessed and so pass intact into the circulation. Because they are antigenic, they stimulate the immunological system, which promptly produces antibodies whose job it is to latch onto the stray bits of protein and remove them from the system. However if there is a defect in the immune system, it can overreact to what under normal circumstances would be perfectly harmless substances and set up a violent inflammatory reaction or allergic response.

There is increasing evidence to suggest that this 'kink' in the immune system — technically known as an immuno-deficiency — which causes excessive production of what are known as IgE antibodies, is inherited and causes a phenomenon known as atopy, a predisposition to hay fever, asthma, migraine and eczema, which may be initiated or exacerbated by common allergens including cows' milk, eggs, wheat products, cat's hair, house dust, feathers, etc. The skin of atopic individuals, especially young children, is notoriously liable to rashes, itchiness, bumps, redness, weeping, and other symptoms of eczema. The whole field of allergy research is a large and complicated one, and immunologists are still trying to fathom out why it is that some individuals should suffer a massive and harmful immune response to what is a perfectly harmless stimulant in the majority of other people and, more to the point, what the precise biochemical mechanism is that triggers the allergic reaction. When it comes to pinning down the offending allergen or food substance, the allergist becomes a clinical detective faced with a formidable array of contradictions and conundrums. Since the majority of eczema patients cannot relate the deterioration of their skin to eating one particular food, many specialists believe that the allergy is probably one of the 'masked' variety, so-called because it is caused by a common foodstuff which is part of a normal everyday diet and therefore, one would think, totally beyond suspicion. Dairy produce, in particular cows' milk and cheese, is thought by many doctors to be a powerful potential allergen, especially in babies and young children whose immune systems are as yet undeveloped, because it is a heavy protein rich in 'strange antigens' and thus takes efficient processing in order to be fully broken down and absorbed in the gut. Doctors stress that breast-fed babies are far less likely to suffer from gastro-intestinal or immunologically-triggered disorders, because compared to bottle feeds based on cows' milk (designed after all for calves not babies) human milk is a natural substance that helps from a very early age to build up and strengthen a baby's immune system and encourage the formation of the right quota of antibodies. Mothers with a history of eczema, or those with a child already suffering from the disease, are particularly encouraged to breast feed in order to minimise the risk of their newborn infants developing eczema and other atopic disorders.

Other common food allergens are wheat-based products (gluten appears to be the offending substance, poorly broken down in the gut), bread, fish, chocolates, eggs, and foods that contain artificial colourings such as tartazine which can also cause outbreaks of nettle rash in some children. Because intradermal prick tests are often useless in identifying the offending food, the best way of finding out whether a person is allergic to a particular food is to exclude it for a trial period of a few weeks and see if the condition improves. By then reintroducing the food after this period and observing how the skin reacts, a so-called 'rotation diet' helps in the process of identifying and confirming which group of foods is to be avoided. Due to much of the excellent scientific work carried out by clinical ecologists on the effects of nutritional and environmental allergens on skin as well as on physical and mental well-being generally, and probably because they make themselves so manifestly obvious, allergies carry a lot more credibility than the concept of deficiencies as a contributory factor to ill health.

One of the most hotly disputed claims is that mental and emotional disturbances and physical symptoms can result from an imbalanced diet, from a lack of certain nutrients caused by the inability of some people to absorb or synthesise certain vitamins and minerals properly. In America, health supplements — vitamins, minerals, herbal extracts, enzymes, etc. — today constitute a billion-dollar industry and Britain is catching up fast, even though the average doctor is scathing in his dismissal of vitamin supplements as a complete waste of money, which can make no difference whatsoever to the person's health. As the polemic flourishes, kicked around between therapy 'nihilists' in the British medical profession who maintain that a good diet solves all, and American-style nutrition therapists who advocate mega-doses of a wide spectrum of nutrients to either cure or fend off every ailment from wrinkles to cancer, evidence that some people may become deficient in some nutrients at some time in their lives, and that this can directly or indirectly affect the health of skin tissue, is growing rather than dwindling. But what constitutes a deficiency in the first place, and what are the criteria used to evaluate a well-balanced, healthy diet?

Health — or Superhealth?

To begin with, some nutritionists maintain that few people recognise what constitutes a truly well-balanced diet in the first place: essentially one rich in green leafy vegetables, fruit, pulses, legumes, whole foods, low-fat dairy produce, and fish, in food eaten as close as possible to its raw natural state, and one that is low in refined foods such as white flour, sugar, saturated fats, alcohol, red meat and other animal protein. Moreover a lot of us are vague about the definition of good health, since we often fail misguidedly to make the distinction between simply not being ill and feeling our very best.

A London nutritionist Barbara Cadwell pulls no punches about optimal health and concludes that migraine, headaches, indigestion, catarrh, insomnia, tiredness, minor depression, aches and pains, persistent spots, pimples, rashes, and fluid retention have no place in the annals of the super health to which we surely all aspire. She maintains that as a result of eating too many refined, processed foods, more and more of us are developing very vague, subtle chemical imbalances — for instance, one in four people has blood sugar problems — which can be traced to faulty eating habits and minor sub-clinical vitamin or mineral deficiencies. What is more, even if and when we eat all the right foods, these may not be tailored to fit a specific lifestyle: anyone who smokes cigarettes and goes on a diet, drinks a lot of alcohol, skips breakfast, takes medication or the contraceptive pill, is under a great deal of stress or suffers from emotional traumas, develops a great dependence on certain nutrients like vitamin C, B-complex vitamins and minerals like zinc, which get used up more quickly by the body. Other therapists like homeopath Michael Van Straten point out that our food is not always as crammed with nutrients as we fondly believe it is. Enzymes and vitamins like C and the B-complex group, both essential for the formation of healthy tissues, nerve fibres and smooth functioning immune systems, are quickly and easily destroyed through processing, storage, heat and light, as well as cooking. Which is why raw vegetables with their cache of life-enhancing enzymes intact are far more nutritious and able to restore and repair the tissues of the body than when they are cooked. Food that is artificially ripened, a common practice among fruit growers, may *look* healthy enough, but its wholesome appearance is largely cosmetic, since the deprivation of sufficient UV light to stimulate full vitamin and mineral synthesis significantly depletes its nutritional value. Intensive 'mono culture' farming methods also strip the soil of trace elements and important minerals such as selenium, which can never be fully restored with artificial fertilisers. Yet even the staunchest advocate of vitamin therapy will agree that vitamin pills are no substitute for healthy eating, but should be regarded instead as an insurance policy against specific weaknesses or used as a back-up at times of stress and llness, and fast track living. Such respected American nutrition-sts as Dr Abraham Hoffer and Dr Roger Williams, Professor of Biochemistry at the University of Texas, far from setting themselves up as self-imposed messiahs of mega-vitamin therapy, have carried out years of intriguing research on both laboratory animals and humans that suggests that it is not how many vitamins you take but what your body does with them that is mportant.

For instance, many people who suffer from serious emotional and mental disturbances seem to lack certain basic enzymes which prevent their bodies from metabolising or adequately processing certain nutrients, impairing or preventing either the synthesis or the absorption of perhaps one or two important vitamins or minerals. Substances that thus veer off target tend to be vitamins B6, B12, pantothenic acid, folic acid, vitamin C and zinc — all essential for the formation of healthy collagen. Even diehard sceptics do not dismiss the 'error theory' out of hand. Indeed geneticists and biochemists are today making the study of congenital defects and how to reverse, prevent and modify their ill effects their life's work, with startling breakthroughs and repercussions in the world of medicine. It is well established, for example, says Dr Joseph Schulman, Professor of Human Genetics at the National Institute of Child Health Development, Bathesda, Maryland, USA, that our metabolism depends for its efficiency on the smooth functioning of our biological machinery whose design was handed down to us with (or without as the case may be) defects and all by our parents, grandparents and great-grandparents. The commonest genetic disease in the world, especially in Greece, Israel and other Mediterranean countries, is the deficiency of a single enzyme (G 6 PD) which affects the metabolism of iron in the red blood cells and causes haemolytic anaemia. Dr Schulman points out that early recognition by a simple blood test is essential, because it is now known that a deterioration of the condition can be held in check by prescribing large doses of vitamin E. G 6 PD is, says Dr Schulman, just one example of an inborn error of metabolism; others result from a deficiency in nutrients like calcium, iron, protein, and a carbohydrate like sugar, while sometimes our requirement for a specific vitamin such as B6, B12 or folic acid (whose deficiency is known to increase the risk of birth defects such as spina bifida in newborn babies) is increased as a result of one of these genetic defects. What emerges clearly therefore is that the whole issue of nutritional supplementation is dependent on the laws of cause and effect — which goes to show that indiscriminately gulping down vast quantities of vitamins from A–Z just to stay fit and healthy is both foolish and a waste of money, and by creating an imbalance could prove potentially harmful.

The best way to make sure that you are getting all the nutrients you need for optimal health and have no in-built dependence on or deficiency of any specific vitamin or mineral is to consult a doctor, nutritional therapist or US-style ortho-molecular therapist, or a practitioner of natural therapies — preferably someone who combines both orthodox and holistic methods — who can conduct certain tests and analyse your diet in relation to your general health and lifestyle.

Vitamin C

Vital to the health of the nervous and immune systems and in maintaining healthy brain and muscle tissue, C is directly involved in the synthesis of collagen and therefore plays an important part in the healing of wounds, burns, bruises, and bleeding gums. Vitamin C also keeps the lining of the blood vessel walls strong and resilient, prevents gums from bleeding and receding, activates the healing of wounds and forms the core or matrix upon which strong healthy bones and teeth are built. As such it is one of the most protective of all vitamins and is closely connected with the smooth function of the white blood cells that fight off infection and the lymph cells of the immune system. A very high concentration of the vitamin is also found in the adrenal glands which gear up the body and provide extra energy at times of stress and physical activity. One recent clinical trial showed that taking extra quantities of C can cause an eighty-three per cent reduction in pressure sores and ulcers, while conversely recovery from skin lesions is delayed through lack of C in the diet, while more ulcers tend to form due to the slowdown of normal connective tissue replacement.

Scurvy, one of the oldest recorded diseases in man and characterised by bleeding gums, loose teeth, loss of hair, and extensive bruising and haemorrhaging of the skin, is the principal symptom of vitamin C deficiency, a link first discovered over 200 years ago when many sailors on long sea voyages died from near zero blood levels of C until consignments of C-rich limes and other citrus fruit were carried aboard to prevent the disease. According to a study carried out by the DHSS in 1979, early clinical signs of scurvy were found to be common in elderly hospital patients, and many doctors stress that people who rely on institutional feeding as for instance in hospitals, schools, and old folks homes, as well as those who are house bound and budget conscious which include the very young, may well run a risk of vitamin C deficiency. That old familiar doctors' dictum that we get all the C we need from half an orange a day is now dismissed by the majority of nutritionists (and remember that doctors as a whole do not study nutrition for any length of time as part of their medical training) as an utterly spurious argument. Our dependence on C goes up at certain times — illness, infection, skin infections and injuries — and the rate at which we use it up can be accelerated by numerous factors.

When you consider the many varied roles that vitamin C has to play in keeping us healthy, nature appears to have short-changed us, in company with monkeys and guinea pigs, considerably. In contrast, scientists have found that it is virtually impossible to induce a vitamin deficiency in laboratory animals such as rats and mice, because of the vast amounts that saturate their tissues — the goat, for example, makes as much as 7 grammes of vitamin C per day! Humans, however, lack the very last enzyme required in the chain that would convert glucose into C in the liver. Unlike other important nutrients such as the B-complex group, physical levels of C are relatively easy to measure in the bloodstream and also in the tissues, since the white blood cell content gives a good indication of blood body levels. Easy monitoring has alerted doctors to the importance of vitamin C in helping the body heal itself and fight off infection. Such precise measurement also illustrates the differing needs of many people and the rate at which they use up the vitamin. For example, when we are under increased stress, extra quantities of the vitamin are promptly pulled out of the tissues and used to protect the body, in turn creating the need for increased intake to meet the demand. Those most at risk are pregnant women, growing children, smokers, heavy drinkers, people on long-term medication, and anyone who is run down and suffering from colds, flu and other infections.

Since vitamin C acts as a detoxifying agent, cigarette smoking not surprisingly has been found to rob the body's store of C at the alarming rate of an estimated 25 mg per cigarette. So obviously anyone smoking ten or twenty cigarettes a day wouldn't do too well on the British RDA (required daily allowance) of 30 mg! Studies carried out at the Karolinska Hospital in Stockholm indicate that in order to keep an adequate supply of this vitamin in the tissues, smokers need to take at least 40 per cent more vitamin C than non-smokers. Alcoholism or heavy drinking depletes the level of every vital nutrient in the body, setting the scene for deficiency symptoms and malnutrition. Yet C is particularly vulnerable because it is used by the body in very large amounts to neutralise and flush alcohol out of the tissues and bloodstream. Indeed massive injections of C are the standard treatment in hospitals for patients admitted in a coma with alcoholic poisoning.

The medicines and daily pills we take also greatly affect our vitamin status, destroying, for example, vitamin C as well as the B-complex range, weakening their theraputic action, or even increasing our need for them. Dr Tapan Basu of the University of Surrey has conducted a comparative study into the blood levels of vitamin C in women using oral contraceptives and found them to be significantly lower than those of other women. A chemical chain-reaction is to blame here, since the hormones used in the Pill create an increase in certain blood proteins, one of which is known to break down the chemical structure of C rendering it inactive. The antiobiotic tetracycline, often used as a long-term anti-acne therapy for teenagers, also interferes with vitamin C as does cortisone, commonly prescribed for indefinite periods to control asthma, arthritis, and eczema. Aspirin has recently been implicated as a prime C scavenger, since it directly inhibits the absorption of the vitamin from the bloodstream by the white blood cells, where it is needed most of all to fight off infection. Probably the most interesting recent discovery is that taking C along with iron-rich foods can increase the body's assimilation of iron quite considerably, thus helping to combat iron deficiency anaemia, a very common symptom amongst women of child-bearing age, which is caused as much by eating insufficient iron in the diet as by not absorbing properly what you do eat. A glass of orange juice (about 70 mg of C) pushes up the body's absorption of iron three-fold, and one and a half glasses will increase it five-fold, but only if taken at the same time and not at separate meals.

Vitamin A

This is essential for maintaining healthy eyesight and strong bones, but the skin is one of the first tissues to be affected by a lack of vitamin A, which causes excessive dryness, flaking, itchiness, and loss of elasticity. Adequate vitamin A is also essential for the healthy growth and repair of the epithelial tissues, the skin and mucus membranes lining the nose, throat, lungs and eyelids. People who are vitamin-A deficient may develop an acne-like condition, as the deepest layers of the skin cells die before they can work their way up to the surface and so the pores of the skin become clogged up with flakes of broken-up dead skin cells, causing an accumulation of cellular debris and secretions and preventing the free flow of skin oils, which eventually leads to infection, pimples and boils. The effect of vitamin A on the epithelial tissues has intrigued scientists ever since the discovery that its deficiency leads to hyperkeratosis — over-activity and fast growth of the outer skin cells — and to changes in the mucus membranes. A recognised feature of precancerous conditions, hyperkeratosis is the common denominator and principal feature in a number of skin diseases, including acne, psoriasis, and rosacea, and although there is as yet no conclusive evidence to suggest that these are necessarily directly associated with A deficiency, the beneficial effects of vitamin A supplements in healing such skin conditions are widespread. The use of the safer, less toxic, retinoids, synthetic vitamin-A derivatives, to treat cystic acne, rosacea, seborrhoea, psoriasis, and certain skin cancers, marks a new and very exciting development in dermatology. Given in very large doses, however, vitamin A is toxic and can cause severe illness and death, which is why the chances of anyone who eats their fair share of vegetables including carrots (the richest source of vitamin A), dairy produce, eggs, or fish and liver, becoming vitamin-A deficient are pretty low. In very large doses vitamin A is toxic because it is stored in the liver to be released over prolonged periods as required. Vitamin A reserves are known to decrease with age and as a result of illness, probably because it is released in large quantities by the liver to help fight infection in the diseased part of the body. For example, because of its depressive action on the body's immune system, one of the commonest side effects of taking cortisone is that wounds or other skin lesions heal very slowly. Research carried out at the University of California showed that when vitamin A was applied directly onto the skin of the patient, their sores healed up within a few days.

Zinc

The relationship between vitamin A and zinc is a very inter-independent one, especially when it comes to collagen synthesis and wound healing: one cannot fully play its role in the production of new collagen without help from the other, and lack of zinc is thought by some scientists in turn to jeopardise levels of vitamin A. Zinc is needed to help the release of A from the liver and to ensure that it is taken up by the tissues. Skin conditions such as psoriasis, acne, and boils, are often found in people with low zinc blood levels, and both oral supplements and zinc ointment for external treatment are used by a number of therapists with considerable success to improve the health of the skin. Zinc deficiency slows down wound healing after surgery, and anyone suffering from burns loses zinc by excretion, running a risk of deficiency and very slow healing. According to Dr Carl Pfeiffer, Director of the Brain Bio-centre in Princeton, New Jersey, women with very low blood levels of zinc run a higher risk of developing stretch marks in pregnancy or as a result of weight gain during puberty, probably because zinc as well as vitamins C and B 6 is needed for effective cross linking of elastin chains to make perfect elastic tissue. Rupture of elastic tissue rather than damaged collagen is responsible for the formation and perma-nent nature of stretch marks.

Scientists believe that today's diet and lifestyle have increased the risk of more people developing zinc deficiency than was thought possible even twenty years ago. Although zinc should ideally be present in many of the foods we eat, there are certain factors which are now known to deplete the mineral quota of many foods and further to inhibit their absorption by the body. Minerals and trace elements come to us principally via the soil on which much of our food is grown, and the characteristics of soil in any particular farming area determine the relative amounts of the elements available for plant and animal life. Certain types of soil may be low or totally deficient in any one trace element, while the availability of certain minerals is determined by antagonism with other minerals present in relatively large amounts. High levels of cadmium in the soil, for example, have an adverse effect on the absorption of zinc from that same soil, while high concentrations of phosphorus inhibit the uptake of zinc and other minerals. Of those minerals which eventually do end up in our food, other factors may inhibit the body's ability to make full use of them. Healthy as a high bran diet undoubtedly is for the condition of the arteries and the cardiovascular system, fibre of all types, and the phytic acid and phosphate present in whole wheat flour, binds up with minerals such as iron and zinc, rendering them unavailable for further use or absorption in the body. A diet rich in calcium and extra high levels of copper in the body are associated with zinc deficiency, while eating mainly processed foods is calculated to depress blood levels of many trace elements including zinc, which are largely destroyed in processing. Illnesses including diabetes, rheumatism, arthritis, lung infections, ulcers, drinking alcohol, too much stress, and taking drugs such as the Pill or cortisone cause a reduction in zinc levels, speeding its excretion in the urine. A dietary supplement of 15/20 mg of zinc a day is sufficient to bolster the body's zinc needs, particularly during recovery from burns, wounds, and other skin lesions.

Selenium

Selenium is another trace element subject to the same vicissitudes as zinc and is extremely low or almost non-existent in the soil of certain parts of the world like England, either because of the excessive use of unbalanced sulphate-based fertilisers or the gradual stripping away by wind and rain. Toxic in high doses, selenium and vitamin E work together synergistically as powerful anti-oxidants, protecting the cells of the body from damage by free radicals. The supply of oxygen-rich blood to the skin and hair tissues is dependent on vitamin E working in conjunction with selenium for optimum effect. Selenium is the only active trace element found in one of the body's most protective anti-ageing enzymes, glutathione peroxidase, a powerful free radical inhibitor, and as such, according to researchers like Dr Richard Passwater, it is a key component of the body's defence against accelerated ageing. Given its pivotal role in guarding the body's cells, it also seems surely no coincidence that in communities where selenium is low the cancer rate is found to be high.

Vitamin E

Like its twin nutrient selenium, vitamin E also has a widespread protective role as an anti-oxidant in body chemistry — the protective enzyme glutathione peroxidase cannot function properly without selenium or vitamin E. The power of vitamin E to heal burns, repair surface wounds, reduce or eliminate the risk of scarring, and shrink pre-existing bunched keloid scars, has been extensively reported, although as yet there is no scientific explanation as to how exactly it speeds tissue healing. Increasing the supply of oxygen to tissues, strengthening of the capillary walls, dilating the small blood vessels, and improving blood flow is, according to researchers, the combined theraputic *modus operandi* of vitamin E. The body's healing process is vitally dependent on constant and adequate sources of oxygen, and patients suffering from severe burns are therefore often exposed to a non-stop stream of sterile oxygen to speed healing. The burns units of a number of hospitals now also use vitamin E, both orally and as a topical ointment, to facilitate this healing process as well as to counteract the formation of ugly bunched scar tissue. Clearly our vitamin E uptake should, along with zinc, vitamin C and selenium, be topped up when the skin is damaged in any way, be it from sunburn, minor cuts and grazes, or serious wounds and burns. Because it is fat-soluble and thus stored in the liver, there is a risk on a day-to-day basis of taking too much E and causing toxic side-effects. A safe dose is between 200–400 international units a day, say nutritionists, which can be built up to 800 units a day for those suffering from skin burns or lesions.

Vitamin F (Essential Fatty Acids)

Widely available in animal fats, vegetables, nuts, and grains, are a group of naturally occurring substances called essential fatty acids, until recently known collectively as vitamin F. These have become the subject of great scientific interest and excitement in biochemists and nutritionists the world over. Those singled out for scrutiny in particular for their importance in helping to maintain healthy skin are linoleic acid, found mostly in seeds and

Maybe
Def

nuts such as sunflower, corn, safflower, sesame, and ground nut, and gamma linoleic acid, which is synthesised in the body from linoleic acid and found only in human breast milk and in oil of evening primrose. Until recently, even nutritionists gave a mere passing nod to the EFAs because it was assumed that since they are prevalent in our high fat diet, a deficiency was unlikely. However, greater research, analysis and understanding of the EFAs, their metabolism in the body and how they are converted into other vital by-products, have led to some fascinating new discoveries about the ways in which the body may become deficient in these substances, despite their presence in the diet. The conversion, for instance, of linoleic acid in the foods we eat into GLA and then into Dihomo-gamma-linoleic acid (DGLA) is an all-important process. For GLA and DGLA are key factors in the manufacture of a group of powerful multi-purpose, hormone-like substances called prostaglandins, whose action in the body is diverse and multifaceted, since they help to regulate inflammatory, blood clotting, hormonal and neurological processes and cholesterol levels. GLA helps to fortify the structure of the membranes that surround all the body's cells, the lipid envelopes surrounding each and every individual cell, and so prevents the skin from losing excess water. Animal experiments show that dry, scaly, ageing skin results when linoleic acid is absent from the diet.

Anyone who eats plenty of vegetable oils (polyunsaturates) would hardly seem a contender for GLA or prostaglandins deficiency, but research shows that the enzymes responsible for converting linoleic acid into GLA are inactivated by factors such as diabetes, viral infections, alcohol, ageing, and a diet high in processed foods, cholesterol and saturated fats, thus blocking the delicate and complex GLA production process. Some people simply labour under an inherited defect that fouls up the enzyme for GLA synthesis, and this defect may also make them more susceptible to certain diseases. Normally stored in the cell membrane ready to be turned into prostaglandins, DGLA reserves are rapidly depleted through heavy drinking and illness, lowering the body's cache of fatty acids even further. Apart from the fact that a diet lacking the whole gamut of essential fatty acids can eventually cause dehydration, scaling, and premature wrinkling of the skin — a distinct danger especially in older people, whose 'draw' on vitamin F is greater yet whose diet is often low in polyunsaturates — red scaly rashes, excessive dryness, and eczema are recognised today as one of the principal features of EFA deficiency, not surprisingly perhaps considering the role of prostaglandins in inflammatory processes.

In one double blind controlled cross-over study reported in the *Lancet* in 1982 by Dr John Burton of the Bristol Royal Infirmary Department of Dermatology, nearly a hundred patients with atopic eczema showed a significant improvement as a result of taking oil of evening primrose, a rich source of GLA and DGLA. Oil of evening primrose has become the subject of worldwide medical trials to establish its effectiveness in treating disorders ranging from skin problems to heart disease, arthritis, multi-sclerosis, and alcoholism. The reason for all the excitement is that this substance neatly side-steps the conversion process of linoleic acid to GLA by providing ready-made GLA which is otherwise only available in human breast milk. According to the last report, the mode of action in eczema sufferers is uncertain, although it is believed to be due to increased manufacture of prostaglandins from the GLA present in evening primrose oil. Eczema sufferers are believed to suffer a genetic deficiency in fatty acids and certain prostaglandins. There is also some evidence to suggest that prostaglandins are involved in the regulation of T-lymphocytes sometimes deficient in people with atopic eczema. Meanwhile, many people taking oil of evening primrose supplement (2×500 mg three times a day) to counteract pre-menstrual tension, eczema, and arthritis, report an improvement in the smoothness and suppleness of their skin, probably because of the ability of LA and GLA to improve the water-binding properties of the skin cells.

To maintain young healthy-looking skin our consumption of EFAs does not have to be excessive, but we should ensure that they come from the best sources — polyunsaturated vegetable and nut oils, and soft margarines like Flora, not *hard* margarines, and processed oils or saturated animal fats like dairy produce and meat — and we should also ensure that nothing interferes with their absorption and mechanism in the body, such as for instance too much alcohol. Researchers stress that certain nutrients like vitamins C and B6, and zinc, are needed in order to protect linoleic acid and help synthesise GLA and prostaglandins correctly, while adequate vitamin E, by preventing the damaging effects of peroxidation, protects all polyunsaturated fatty acids from being destroyed and attacked once they have become incorporated into the fatty cell membranes.

Inner Pollutants

Alcohol

Apart from the potentially devastating and deadly havoc it can wreak on general physical and mental well-being, excessive amounts of alcohol taken regularly or over prolonged periods are particularly noxious for anyone suffering from rosacea, rhyno-phyma (rosacea and swelling of the nose), chronic facial redness, or a tendency to broken capillaries. The reasons for this are quite obvious. Alcohol raises the blood pressure, widens the blood vessels, makes the capillary walls more fragile and liable to rupture, and stimulates the flow of blood to the skin. In normal circumstances, this might result in slight temporary flushing, but in someone with weak and already dilated capillary walls and a tendency to heightened circulation the effect is to heap insult upon injury and create permanent damage to the blood vessels, dilating and rupturing their walls even further.

Damage to blood vessels is only one part of the story, for neither is the coarse, leathery, dehydrated and deeply lined complexion a coincidental affliction of heavy drinkers. In order to metabolise alcohol, the liver manufactures certain enzymes which convert alcohol into a chemical called acetaldehyde, a powerful free radical which, if present in very large quantities in the long term, poses a formidable threat to the tissues as a cross linking agent. Dehydration, wrinkles, loss of elasticity, and a coarse dull skin surface, are part of the same alcoholic legacy that results in hardening of the arteries, brain and liver damage, and birth defects in unborn children. Worse still, long-term heavy alcohol abuse can damage the liver to the point where it is no longer able to produce enough of the enzymes necessary to remove acetaldehyde from the system. It is the steady accumulation of this chemical, not of alcohol itself, which is in fact responsible for the ravages to brain and body tissues alike due to over-drinking.

Puffiness of the tissues, coarsening of the skin texture, surface dryness, and deepening of lines and wrinkles is also due to the short-term side-effect of dehydration following excessive alcohol intake — similar changes can be seen in the skin after long-distance air travel and are part and parcel of jet lag, a syndrome largely aggravated through dehydration.

Smoking

That smoking is a major health hazard which can cause premature deaths from cancer, emphysema, lung disease, and heart attack, is a long and well-established fact with which few people would take issue today. Less drastic are the effects of cigarette smoking on skin tissue, but they are well worth considering if you care about preserving the youth and smoothness of your complexion for as long as possible. Dermatologists maintain that smokers screw up their eyes and frown and pout more as a part of the smoker's repertoire of facial mannerisms that accompany inhalation, exhalation and drawing on a cigarette, stippling and cross-hatching the face with extra and premature lines and wrinkles. But there are two more reasons why the skin of heavy smokers often appears coarser, dryer, and more lined than that of non-smokers.

Oxygen exists at a premium in the tissues and bloodstream of the smoker; its level is depleted as noxious gases from cigarette smoke, carbon monoxide, nitrogen oxides, and our old bogie acetaldehyde, stage a subtle *coup d'etat* within the body, sabotaging the oxygen-carrying capacity of the bloodstream. Not only do the tissues become starved of oxygen and thus of vital cell nutrients, but these toxic-free radicals get to work, damaging the structure of the body's proteins and nucleic acids and causing subtle and insidious destructive influences and changes within the tissues that lead to cross linkage of collagen and elastic fibres. In order to neutralise these toxic chemical pollutants before they can have any serious impact on the body, vitamin C is pulled out of the tissues at a far faster rate and in greater quantities than normal, leaving a deficit which unless it is regularly replaced can impair the process of new collagen formation. Extra quantities of zinc, selenium, vitamins E, A, and B6 as well as vitamin C can also help to prevent the damaging effects of oxidation and free radicals within the body generally.

Sleep and Exercise

We all know that when we go without deep, restful sleep for any length of time, our skin, especially on the face, is the first area to show the deficit in the form of dull tone, coarse texture, slackness, lines of tension, worry, and fatigue, and a generally 'lifeless' quality. But what is certainly less well known is that there seems to be a certain scientific logic behind it all. The cells of the skin, as well as other surface tissues, divide in a circadian rhythm (which has been observed by watching cell division under lab conditions and counting radioactively labelled cells to measure cell replication) and in adult humans, cells reproduce themselves most actively between midnight and 4 a.m., the time when most of us are asleep. Scientists believe that all this action may be due to a surge of hormones and other metabolic changes that occur during sleep.

Similarly, studies show that vigorous exercise does more for the skin than just make it glow by stimulating the flow of blood and supply of oxygen to its surface tissues. Though that's certainly part of the picture. According to studies carried out on ex-Olympic athletes in Finland — some of whom remained active while others gave up exercising — regular, vigorous exercise seems to accelerate cell division and improve collagen and other protein synthesis, thereby measurably thickening the dermis and preventing premature, degenerative changes. When exercise was stopped, however, these improvements were found to diminish, along with fitness levels.

At the University of Pennsylvania Medical School, Dr Albert Kligman has conducted research using hamsters which he classifies as 'very nervous, active, type A individuals, who thrive on life in the fast track'. The hamsters were kept active — and presumably quite happy — trotting around all day on spinning wheels and other contraptions and then confined to a relatively inactive state. Within less than eight weeks their skin had atrophied, thinned, dried out, and acquired other classic symptoms of premature ageing. Dr Kligman believes that collagen and other connective tissue proteins form a reservoir which can be continuously topped up with vigorous activity, but the source soon becomes dried out when we cease to exercise regularly — as witnessed by the degenerative changes in the skin tissue of hospital patients of all ages who are confined to bed for any length of time after leading a previously active life. Dr Kligman hopes to turn his attention now from hamsters to hospital patients in an attempt to substantiate further his claims that a good fitness programme brings very positive benefits to the appearance and 'lasting power' of skin.

Stress and Emotional Conflict

Skin is a mirror of the psyche: when stress, nervous tension, emotional trauma, anxiety, and a host of related conditions affect our lives, sooner or later our skin is bound to come out in sympathy, for it does not readily withhold much information about the battles waged deep beneath its surface. And why should it? From conception our nervous system and skin are closely related. It is thought that as the spinal cord begins to develop, its cells divide outwards to build skin tissue and thereafter the two systems remain at this almost identical stage of foetal growth. In the embryo, the nerves and skin develop simultaneously and are derived from the same foetal cells. Both types of cells share a very similar biochemistry when it comes to damage and repair mechanism, and are stimulated to grow by structurally very similar hormones.

Skin has also been described by many a psycho-sexual researcher as one vast primary erogenous zone offering, in the right circumstances, a continuum of erotic sensations varying according to area, stimulus, mood and individual. The pride and pleasure that we take in exposing and even decorating, through jewellery, fashions and cosmetics, our own skin, can greatly determine its receptivity to touch and affect the development of our tactile senses, not only during lovemaking and sexual enjoyment but as a part of our everyday life and well-being. This in turn may profoundly affect our sensuality, self-confidence, and ability to participate in and to enjoy sex, as well as to express love and affection generally through touch and other forms of non-verbal communication. Skin carries over five billion sensory nerve cells programmed, at the right touch, to send messages to the brain to initiate sexual activity. Receptors trigger arousal, especially in the genital region and the erogenous zones rich in nerve fibres, such as the breasts, thighs, feet, and back, sending further feedback to the central nervous system resulting in sexual excitement and orgasm.

The sensitivity of body tissue and its receptivity to touch and other stimuli can fluctuate immensely, not just in different areas, different people, and at different ages and periods of a person's life, but more subtly and rhythmically as a result of the hormonal changes that perpetuate a woman's menstrual cycle. Many women become more acutely sensitive and tuned-in to erotic skin sensations, feel sexier, and alternately more aggressive or passive at various stages within each month. For example, during ovulation, combined high oestrogen and progesterone levels may have the effect of giving an extra-sensory 'edge' to the erectile tissues of the breasts and clitoris, fuelling sexual desire and heightening receptivity, while pre-menstrual fluid retention, provided it is not too extreme or uncomfortable, congests the tissues of the labia, vulva, and clitoris, and makes the breasts fuller and more sensitive and responsive to touch, adding a whole constellation of erotic trimmings to sexual encounters as well as to even the most casual and fleeting forms of body contact. In certain cases, taking drugs can mimic this sensory high — although certain women experience a blunting of tactile, erotic sensation when drinking alcohol or experimenting with mari-huana or cocaine, a drug usually recognised for its potential in increasing sexual enjoyment and sharpening sensory perception.

Like litmus paper skin vividly and rapidly records shifting frissons of excitement and emotion. Anger and fear drain blood from the tissues and turn us pale; hostility tightens the muscles, while lines of hardness and tension cleave into the facial contours; embarrassment flushes the complexion, neck and chest, and makes the skin shiny; anxiety causes us to break out in a sweat; sexual arousement, orgasm makes every inch of the body skin tingle and glow. These involuntary responses, governed by the sympathetic branch of the body's autonomic nervous system, over which we have little or no control, offer fleeting yet incontestable evidence of the skin's involvement along with the heart, muscles, digestive organs, and blood vessels in the body's 'fight or flight' response to stress.

Links and Pathways

Defined by the late father of stress research Dr Hans Selye as a three-phase 'specific adaptation syndrome', the initial stage of stress is one of alarm: the hypothalmus, aided and abetted by its number two, the pituitary gland, sends finely coordinated messages to the adrenal glands which then pump a massive output of stress hormones including adrenalin, noradrenalin, and cortisone into the system. The immediate effect of these chemicals is to increase the heart rate, raise the blood pressure, body temperature and oxygen consumption, release cholesterol from the liver, and shunt the flow of blood away from vital organs towards the brain, shutting off digestion and tensing the muscles. Thus revved up into a state of arousal, this welter of activity heralds the second resistance stage as the body struggles to maintain homeostasis, its normal state of inner balance. It is at this crucial point that our individual reactions to stress manifest themselves, because the main force of the pressure is usually directed at one particular target area within the body which must then go into a state of overdrive, pulling out all the stops to adapt itself to the upheaval. In one person the stomach may be the prime stress site, in another the heart and connecting arteries, in someone else the immune system may react adversely, setting off attacks of asthma, hay fever and skin disorders such as eczema, psoriasis, etc. Not surprisingly perhaps, the more effectively a particular organ or system adapts to stress, the more likely it eventually will be to malfunction and weaken. This marks the final exhaustion phase when that part of the body breaks down altogether. Alarming though these reactions may sound, our bodies are of course superbly well equipped to cope with stress —indeed some of us seem to thrive on it. We are often told that one man's stress is another man's stimulus, but the point is for how long? We all know that we can run many different electrical appliances off one power circuit for a certain period, but that once we overload the system it will break down, blowing a fuse. Few of us would dispute this analogy with human stress or strain; indeed as one leading researcher points out, if we were to subject an electrical system to as much abuse and pressure as we do our bodies, we would probably spend over half our lives in a perpetual blackout! Dr Selye refers to such widespread stress-related ailments as ulcers, diabetes, hypertension, heart disease, and asthma as 'diseases of adaptation', a theory which in recent years has helped to illustrate the diversity of human reactions to stress.

Mind Over Matter

Anyone who has experienced flushes, rashes, itchiness, and swelling of the skin, not to mention the more physically debilitating and alarming pains of the stress syndrome when it reaches chronic proportions, knows how physically and emotionally depleting it is. The most sinister aspect of stress is, however, its insidiousness, which explains why many people agonise and fret over chronic or recurrent skin problems which appear to have *no* underlying physical cause, unable to recognise these as the symptoms of long-term, persistent and accumulated stress. For there is absolutely no doubt that stress can prove as corrosive to your appearance as to your general health — indeed one is usually the effect of the other. Indirectly, the effects of prolonged and persistent stress on the nervous system and organs can trap the body in a vicious stress spiral, opening up a Pandora's box of major and minor symptoms including acne, eczema, cellulite, weight gain or extreme weight loss, premature ageing, herpes, psoriasis, and pigmentation disorders, linked to the effects of emotional trauma on the immune system. The skin after all is directly dependent for its good health and appearance on all the other glands in the body, in particular the thyroid, ovaries, pituitary, and adrenals, and is therefore subject to the vagaries of the brain's hypothalmus master gland and the pituitary, which may, under stress, upset the finely synchronised mechanism of the body's hormone production.

It has been established that over a third of all patients who consult a dermatologist have emotional problems that are, to one degree or another, the cause of their skin disorder. In a competitive career woman who also runs a home and a family, scalp problems, hair loss, and acne may be the direct result not only of muscular tension and the excess production of adrenalin and other stress chemicals, but of a gradual elevation of the levels of the male sex hormone testosterone which acts as a fuel to aggressive, competitive behaviour, perpetuating a stressful life-style. Over-secretion of testosterone in some people triggers sebaceous activity and hair loss. According to leading trichologist Philip Kingsley, his trichological clinics in New York and London have in just the last few years treated 25 per cent more women for problems of hair loss and thinning than ever before. These disorders he believes are attributable to the rise in stress factors and nervous tension in the lives of young working women. Because the exact mechanism that causes eczema, psoriasis, pigmentation disorders, and even acne still remains unknown, the treatments prescribed by doctors are symptom-oriented and so by their nature tend to be suppressive or palliative. No self-respecting doctor would ever dream of talking about a 'cure' for acne or psoriasis since, strictly speaking there is none.

In tune with the prevailing 'holistic' ethos that shapes the field of alternative medicine, skin ailments — along with organic disfunction, chronic aches and pains, and emotional disturbances — are rarely treated as an isolated symptom. Establishing the root cause of the skin problem, whether its origins stem from physical imbalance or psychological conflict, is what counts in successful therapy. Interestingly enough, dermatology is one area of medicine where conservatism has undergone a volte-face in recent years, and an increasing number of specialists faced with skin disorders that remain unresponsive to orthodox medicine, will nowadays refer patients to an alternative practitioner, conceding that some chronic complaints may well be largely in the mind. The results of alternative therapy are often spectacular. Mandy Langford is a London-based hypnotherapist who has specialised in treating and curing men, women and children for psychosomatic skin disorders, many of them what she calls medical 'rejects', referred by doctors and dermatologists in a last-ditch attempt at successful treatment when all else has failed. Chronic disorders like eczema, psoriasis, spots, pimples and rashes have, she observes, their origins in very early childhood trauma and the automatic repression of painful emotional experiences which turns those feelings inwards and right back into the subconscious, only to erupt in the form of emotional stress-linked skin ailments later in life. Laboratory studies have established that in eczema-prone individuals, emotional arousal increases the amount of fluid secreted by the skin cells while relaxation diminishes it. Similarly, teenagers suffering from acne have been found to suffer more severe outbreaks of the disorder just before and during sitting exams.

Unravelling the Past

The hidden pathways connecting psyche and skin are by no means easy to locate. Troubled emotions flare up in the guise of rashes, blemishes, and any manner of sores, either with infuriating unpredictability or tedious regularity, bridging a synapse of time and self-deception. Therefore any experience, event, or stressful occasion, that, however subconsciously, kindles early suppressed feelings of anxiety, fear, guilt, or shame may act as a catalyst in the outbreak of a skin complaint. The greatest value of hypnotherapy lies in its power to locate and identify not only the existing stress factors in a person's life that make him or her likely candidates for skin disorders, but, more important, the deep-rooted, suppressed emotions, conflicts and neuroses that lie embedded in the subconscious. Through exorcising the latter, therapists like Mandy Langford are able not only to remove distressing and disabling skin disorders for good, but to enhance an individual's emotional and mental well-being by helping him or her to understand and resolve psychic 'angst' and pain. Not that hypnotherapy offers a fast or magic cure for rashes and blemishes, let alone psychological malaise. Therapy consists of three distinct stages. The primary goal is to tackle the immediate source of stress in a person's life which appears linked to the outbreaks of eczema, acne, psoriasis, etc. Deep-relaxation techniques and hypnosis can help a person control excessive stress and pressure at work, cope with discord within domestic life or a personal relationship, and unravel sexual hangups. The clue here lies in assessing how patients feel on an emotional level and why they experience these feelings whenever they develop a rash. At this stage the main aim is to help patients to 'get in touch' with often suppressed or ignored feelings. Anger, guilt, fear, lack of self-esteem, and panic, are some of the commonest suppressed emotions which become channelled or sublimated through the skin, usually at times of strife and trouble between parents, lovers, spouse, or authoritative figures at work, or during an upheaval such as marriage, engagement, divorce, death, moving house, changing career, redundancy, facing promotion, etc.

Having identified the psychological factors germane to their skin disease and helped patients recognise, and if possible control, the concomitant stresses and strains, the next step is 'transference' of the actual rash under hypnosis from one part of the body to another where the disfigurement is less distressingly conspicuous. A rash on the face may be shifted down to say the ankles or feet, scaly patches transmitted from the fingers to the back of the knees. The temptation to remove the disease completely before working on the underlying cause must be avoided at all costs, since it is only likely to recur in a far worse form. The final stage and the one that is most challenging and can take longest to resolve is the 'diagnostic scan', which consists of regressing patients, taking them back under hypnosis to that point in their lives when they first manifested the feelings of anxiety or shock which have remained suppressed and unresolved. As with most people who undergo psychotherapy for emotional disorders, phobias, or obsessive-compulsive behaviour patterns, the time of treatment, especially at this crucial stage of therapy before patients can get in touch with their innermost feelings and learn to control or channel them productively, depends largely on the nature and severity of the underlying emotional block as well as on the trust and rapport that exists between therapist and patient. Skin disorders must be treated within the context of a person's life, and therapists such as Mandy Langford eschew limited goals — a fast but temporary recovery from the skin disorder — in favour of in depth healing of both mind and skin. This can take time, but it inevitably yields a catharsis that not only benefits a person's appearance and visceral well-being, but may profoundly revolutionise the way that he or she leads their life. Mandy Langford has found that women with chronic psychosomatic skin diseases, just like people who are chronic nail-biters or compulsive over-eaters, or those with a drink problem, are very often victims of a panoply of predominately 'female' anxieties that undermine their self-esteem and self-confidence. Sexual fears and inhibitions are often the underlying problem in young women, as is the need for approval from others to 'sanctify' their self-image and inspire feelings of worth; sensations of helplessness, hopelessness and victimisation, and not having control over one's life are, say therapists, often the psychological building blocks behind a mosaic of skin disorders.

The increasing number of patients who visit a psychotherapist or hypnotherapist with chronic or acute skin problems affords further evidence of the tremendous power exerted by the mind over physical well-being and disease. Although hypnotherapy seems a well-accepted and successful mode of treatment for psychologically-oriented skin disorders, excellent results and all-out cures for persistent stress-linked acne, psoriasis and eczema, as well as warts and chronic skin problems, are also reported by people who have studied meditation and creative imagery, which combines deep-relaxation techniques with powerful mental 'imaging'. These exercises involve visualising that part of the skin or body that is diseased and imagining the disease under attack from the body's immune system or from some other healing force, then visualising the skin as it would look in its perfect, unblemished state. Other exercises which involve altered states of consciousness are based on a verbal dialogue with the diseased part of the skin in order to secure its eventual disappearance. Much as many people might deride or dismiss such unconventional healing methods as so much hocus-pocus, the crackpot leanings of the lunatic fringe, to dismiss these alternative therapies and their exponents out of hand is to turn a blind eye to the very real benefits, remissions, and inexplicable miracle cures that hundreds of sufferers from everything from cancer to eczema have derived as a result of following such lines of treatment. Belief in the system of choice may have much to do with the response of the body — the so-called 'placebo response' is as powerful and prevalent a healing factor in holistic medicine as it is in orthodox medicine. Certainly as far as non-life-threatening skin diseases go, there is no health hazard, nothing to be lost and everything to be gained by undergoing alternative treatments even as a first line of choice.

Electrical Feedback

Because of the electrical charge present in each of its millions of cells, the skin's ever changing patterns of electrical activity offer one of the most easily measurable and instant and accurate monitoring systems of mental and physical harmony and discord. How rapidly and intensely the autonomic nervous system becomes aroused in reaction to stress and how promptly and automatically the 'fight or flight' response is quietened down by its opposite number, the relaxation response, which is activated by the para-sympathetic branch of the nervous system, can be measured by changes in the skin's electrical properties. As far back as 1905 Carl Jung demonstrated the correlation between physical arousal and changes in electrical skin resistance, but today highly refined and sophisticated electronic biofeedback equipment has been developed, which is so sensitive to this ionic interplay within the epidermis that it can accurately quantify levels of skin stress by measuring precisely every notch on the vast scale of physical arousal, from general anaesthesia or catatonia at one end of the spectrum to extreme panic states at the other. Such biofeedback machinery, along with more sophisticated equipment that measures the fluctuations in brain wave patterns during states of stress and relaxation, is proving an invaluable therapeutic tool in combating stress-related illnesses or as an adjunct to meditation and deep-relaxation techniques, since these provide both therapist and patient with a valuable instant guide to a person's current levels and patterns of arousal, and the ability to control these patterns and relax.

The galvanic skin arousal meter has proved a reliable tool in the instant diagnosis of latent mental and physical disorders. Basal skin readings taken at random may show 'slow arousal' — a symptom of impending nervous crisis, chronic fatigue, anxiety, tension, and depression. An increase in electrical skin resistance indicates the complete opposite of stress and is accompanied by a decrease in oxygen intake, lowered heart and respiratory rate, and a drop in blood pressure, muscle tone, adrenalin, cholesterol and cortisone levels. Biofeedback, which is used increasingly by hospitals to treat people suffering from hypertension, works by emitting differing signals — usually via a bleep, flashing light, or a needle on a dial — which attest to a person's current state of physical tension or relaxation. By learning to control and decode these messages and modulate the frequencies associated with 'uptightness' emitted by the skin, biofeedback helps people to tune in to their own stress levels and learn how to control them more easily. The actual mechanism of changes in the skin's resistance is a fiendishly complex one. Variables that affect the skin's resistance are eating a very heavy meal, alcohol, smoking, taking drugs, whether the time of reading is night or day, and especially anxiety and fatigue. When we are under stress, physical arousal is accompanied by a constriction in the blood vessels beneath the skin's surface and a drop in blood flow to the tissues, and therefore electrical skin resistance is decreased, while conversely, higher skin resistance reflects dilation of the capillaries and increased blood flow, and therefore indicates that the body is relaxed. By succinctly spelling out how smoothly or erratically we veer between alternative states of arousal and relaxation, the electrical language of skin provides an eloquent reminder of the all-pervasive, hidden hazards of stress.

CHAPTER 11
The Neglected Areas

Turn skin inside out and we soon perceive its beauty is far from confined to the outer surface. Take a long hard look at its sum square footage and it soon becomes obvious that skin care goes way beyond jaw level, even though most of us seem predominantly obsessed with the facial tissues, trusting to chance and good luck and leaving the rest of our body skin to fend largely for itself. Which it will, to a certain degree and up to a certain age, after which discomfort and flaws will eventually force us to become more aware of those giveaway areas of neglect. Though patch-up salvage operations are no substitute for regular, all-over body care, it is never too late to rectify some of the damage incurred, and the difference it could mean to both the comfort and appearance of the body generally may prove phenomenal.

Legs

Swollen puffy legs and varicose veins are twin afflictions that face most men and women alike at some stage or other in their lives. The problem of puffiness and swelling can range from mild and transient, be caused by long-distance air travel, spending very long periods standing up, and walking for long periods on concrete pavements, to the more chronic oedema that accompanies or heralds pre-menstrual tension, kidney disorder, a sedentary life-style, hormonal imbalances, or weight gain. Barring any serious underlying organic cause, swelling in the legs can be alleviated by cutting down salt in the diet — salt promotes fluid retention — or by taking a mild diuretic, especially in the case of pre-menstrual fluid retention, by wearing support tights or stockings to minimise strain and pressure on the veins, by sitting or lying down with the legs raised and supported as high off the floor as possible, and by avoiding standing around for too long. Splashing or plunging the legs alternately into warm or cool water also helps to reduce tenderness or swelling by stimulating the flow of circulation. Varicose veins, to which chronic swelling and congestion of the tissues are often a precurser, affects over five million people in Britain and a greater percentage of women than men. Although obesity, pregnancy, lack of exercise, and constipation are often precipitating or exacerbating factors in the development of varicose veins, hereditary weakness of the walls of the veins ultimately determines whether someone is a sufferer. Bumpy, hard or marblised veins, general swelling, soreness, tiredness and heaviness in the legs, as well as bouts of cramp, are early warning signs that the valves in the vein which open and shut automatically to allow blood to course through and prevent back-flow have become faulty and ceased to work efficiently. The result? Blood flow is held back, pushing, stretching and clogging up the valve below. If the veins are isolated and small, they can be shut off through the injection of a sclerosing fluid which causes the blood to clot inside them, but when a long or entire section of the saphenous vein which runs from the groin to the inner ankle or the short saphenous that travels from the back of the knee to the outer ankle, is involved, surgery may be necessary to remove the vein altogether through a procedure known as 'stripping'. Bluish, bruised-looking, spidery surface veins or spider neavi are not in any way indicative of varicose veins, and since they lie near the surface of the skin these can be faded through injections of sclerosing fluid, sodium tetradecyl sulphate, or the use of a CO_2 laser to dry up the blood within the distended and/or ruptured capillaries.

Cellulite

The British medical profession sceptically dismiss cellulite — those wads of hard, dimpled flesh on the upper thighs and buttocks — as a fancy foreign pseudonym for ordinary fat, a fashionable piece of hokum dreamt up by beauticians and cosmetic companies to justify the exorbitant costs of a wide variety of spot slimming treatments and products. Fat, say doctors, is fat, even if merely manifested in isolated plaques on the thighs on someone who is otherwise slim and not overweight and who eats moderately and exercises regularly. But French and Italian doctors have, on the contrary, long isolated some unique characteristics that identify cellulite and set it apart as a phenomenon quite different from the surplus fat of the upper body. To begin with, cellulite unlike fat is essentially a woman's disorder, men do not suffer from it; moreover it is a problem seen very often on women who are slim or of otherwise normal proportions and weight.

Unlike ordinary fat, cellulite is always localised and mainly confined to the lower half of the body, gravitating towards the upper thighs — that famous 'riding breeches bulge' that ruins the line of trousers, tight skirts, leotards, and swim suits — the buttocks, the inside and tops of knees. Either the flesh is hard, lumpy and pitted, with an uneven, shadowy and corrugated-looking surface, or the skin, when pinched, looks dimpled, and a mass of tiny hard nodules can be felt underneath which roll like grains of rice under pressure from the edge of the thumb. It is those fatty nodules, say French doctors, that distinguish cellulite from neighbouring fat on the tummy, waist, arms, hips, etc., which is almost always smooth and uniform. Cellulite does not disappear or even greatly improve with dieting and exercise, and it can be masked initially by surface fat and therefore remain undiagnosed until, paradoxically, weight has been lost.

The reason why cellulite seems indigenous to the female population is because nature has lumbered us with unfair twin handicaps in the first place: hormonal fluctuations *and* an extra quota of fatty tissue which distinguishes the female from the male physique. Women *do* carry more fat, and those surplus layers are laid down chiefly in the pelvic region, the hips and thighs, but over and above those extra fat cells cellulite has compex links with the pituitary master gland which regulates hormonal activity and in particular the cyclical ebb and flow of oestrogen, one of the prime catalysts in the formation of cellulite because of its links with fluid retention. This is why cellulite is more likely to appear or worsen at puberty, ovulation, pre-menstrually, during pregnancy, or at any time when the delicate machinery of the hormonal cycle is upset by stress, illness or shock, or major biological change.

Cellulite has been defined by European doctors and endocrinologists as an extreme and chronic manifestation of poor circulation, impaired lymphatic drainage, and fluid retention. Dr

Phillip Frost of Miami's Mount Sinai Hospital, who has carried out extensive studies into the causes of cellulite, points out that the different ways in which fat is 'laid down' in men and women probably account for this uniquely female phenomenon. Not only do we have more fat cells than men, but our surface skin is thinner and the connective fibres that divide up fat tissue and hold it in place are laid down in a more irregular pattern which pushes the fat into thick uneven globules, giving the skin on the upper thighs and buttocks a pitted or bumpy mattress effect when pinched. Men's fatty tissue, on the other hand, is arranged in a neater, more symmetrical fashion, so that the fat is held firmly in shape giving the most over-blown beer gut a smooth uniformity! Professor Marks of the Welsh National School of Medicine in Cardiff describes cellulite as 'an anatomical derangement due to the shape of the individual'. It is localised, collective and fat tissue which many women are born with and which becomes more noticeable with time. But isn't that perhaps an overly simplistic explanation? According to other research, factors which trigger circulatory upsets are general stress, muscular nervous tensions, severe emotional shock or trauma, faulty diet, lack of exercise, bad posture, and any accident however slight that alters the structure of the spine, lumbar region, legs or feet, and it is important, say those therapists who have been treating cellulite successfully for many years in France and Britain, that all these factors are taken into consideration and that the patient is thoroughly examined for any such imbalances prior to embarking on treatment. To date any foreign reports and findings on the nature of cellulite have been dismissed as contentious by British doctors, and instead of conducting any research or proffering an alternative theory which might invalidate the findings of their foreign counterparts, they seem content merely to dig their heels in and let the matter rest unresolved.

Whatever the pathological differences between 'obesity type' fat and cellulite, one thing seems certain: according to current research on the Continent it seems that the condition can only be improved and even sometimes elimated by controlling and eliminating the basic causes of sluggish circulation and lymph drainage, and hormonal imbalance. This means tracing the stress factors and emotional traumas in a patient's life, evaluating the connection between, say, pre-menstrual tension and the use of the contraceptive pill, reviewing a woman's diet — certain foods *do* cause the body to retain fluid more readily — and making sure that the sufferer drinks six to eight large glasses of water or herbal tea a day to activate the kidneys and aid the elimination of surplus fluid. A sedentary lifestyle or a job that keeps a woman standing around for hours on end is certainly liable to encourage poor circulation as well as allowing the buttock and thigh muscles to become weak and flabby, making cellulite appear worse. While exercise invariably helps to burn up calories and prevents them from turning into fat, the type of activity suitable for slimming the thighs and bottom is fundamentally quite different from that needed to exercise the heart and lungs and cultivate stamina. Any exercise for instance which overworks and builds up the leg muscles or jars the lower joints is unsuitable for anyone doing battle with cellulite. So try and avoid jogging or running; ballet dancing, keep fit or conditioning exercises are excellent, because they have been tailored to elongate and tone up the legs without strain. Avoid vigorous games like tennis and squash which, because they are competitive, raise the body's stress levels. Fast walking is about the best activity, followed by swimming, cycling and yoga.

As with all common figure and skin problems, prevention is a far more formidable weapon against cellulite than any exotic cure so far invented. For the past couple of decades French beauty therapists have capitalised, at times unashamedly, on women's obsession with slimming down their thighs and hips in order to appear fashionably boyish in tight trousers and bikinis. Consequently, the wide choice of costly anti-cellulite treatments available today are sometimes as bewildering as they are grossly misleading, for, contrary to the claims, there is no pill, injection, machine, serum or cream which will magically melt away or break up fat deposits over a short space of time. So-called anti-cellulite treatments, however, do often produce very favourable results by helping to firm and tighten the body muscles of the lower half of the body, improving localised circulation, metabolising waste matter, and toning up and smoothing the skin, provided intensive massage forms an integral part of the treatment. This is why the use of the G5 electronic massage machine or any very intensive hand massage can greatly help to smooth out localised deposits of surplus fat and fluid on the hips, thighs and buttocks. But first check up with your doctor to establish whether you are suffering from a possible hormonal imbalance.

This can prove a valuable indication as to the true nitty-gritty of the problem. If you are generally prone to pre-menstrual physical changes or are going through a phase of hormonal upheaval, this might in itself cast light on the situation.

Scalp

Like spots and pimples, dandruff in any of its many forms, from major, unsightly and chronic to mild, transient and largely unnoticeable, is something that most men and women experience at some time or another in their lives. But it is a ubiquitous umbrella term often used to cover the gamut of scaly disorders from mild or moderate flaking of the scalp a few days after shampooing, to the severe scaling and enflamed patches on the skin, accompanied by over-active oil glands, which constitute seborrheic dermatitis.

Scalp problems are often, by their very nature, an extension of a general skin or facial problem, as in the case of extreme greasiness during adolescence, psoriasis, eczema, and fungus infections such as ringworm. More serious scaly disorders should all be diagnosed and treated by a dermatologist or a trichologist. Exactly what causes dandruff remains a mystery, although stress, faulty diet and illness, through the chemical changes they trigger in the body, may increase cell turnover thus causing flakiness while accelerating sebaceous activity and altering the pH level of the normal scalp secretions. Dandruff is, however, *not* catching, contrary to popular belief, nor is it a sign of lax hygiene. In fact shampooing frequently with very harsh antiseptic anti-dandruff products, often far too abrasive and packed with strong man-made chemicals designed to eliminate greasiness, can wreak havoc with a scalp already tender and sensitive through inflammation, excessive cell turnover and itching. Insult is therefore added to injury when the harsh chemical products get to work on the skin, drying out the surface, and irritating and inflaming the area even further. Regular washing with a mild shampoo helps to control excess greasiness, however, dislodges loose flakes of scalp skin, and keeps the hair itself looking clean, shiny, and free from scales. If irritation and soreness persist, a dermatologist or tricologist may prescribe a special treatment shampoo and lotion based on zinc, salicylic acid, tar, and selenium sulphide, to help dislodge the build-up of sticky scales and control the bacteria and yeast organisms which aggravate scalp tissues causing inflammation. When choosing over-the-counter scalp and hair products it may be a matter of trial and error to hit on one that is effective enough to control a bad case of dandruff without brutalising the skin and thus perpetuating the condition. 'Dry' dandruff, which consists of a very fine powdery fall of scalp particles and a dry scalp and hair with no hint of oiliness, is far easier to control by using a bland creamy shampoo designed for dry hair and further treating the scalp with a conditioner. The drier the scalp and the more liable it is to inflammation, tenderness, and redness, the more advisable it is to steer clear of any treatments — perming, tinting, bleaching — which use very powerful harsh chemicals. The use of heated rollers, curling tongs, and very hot hair dryers, which may all further scratch and aggravate the scalp, should be kept to a minimum.

Lesser known dandruff-like scalp disorders

Pityriasis amiantacea: An asbestos-like 'clinging vine' of scales builds up along the hair shaft and can cause hair loss if allowed to go untreated. Once cured the hair grows back normally.

Psoriasis: Scales are identical to those on other parts of the body — red patches with silver-white surface scales. Though the scales, if unattractive, are not as itchy or irritating as ordinary dandruff, psoriasis of the scalp still needs attention and treatment to bring the problem as much as possible under control, remembering, however, that there is no sure-fire cure for this skin disorder, which can go through periods of spontaneous remission, and become exacerbated through stress, shock, and illness.

Ringworm: A fungus infection appears on the scalp as whitish scaly patches prone to baldness or thinning of the hair. The disorder can be cured with systemic anti-fungal therapy.

Atopic eczema: This may be due to one of a multitude of allergens or irritants (notably the chemicals and metals used in hair processing and styling techniques), in which case it is technically known as contact dermatitis. Extremely itchy, these red raw patches can 'weep', and become inflamed, damp and encrusted. Treatment may consist of topical corticosteroid creams or ointments or bland soothing lotions to calm down the inflammation and reduce soreness. Ideally, prevention is the best way of curing eczema of the scalp and avoiding a recurrence.

Discoid lupus erythematosis: This usually shows up as reddish-brown scaly patches accompanied by hair loss and 'plugged' hair follicles. It can be cured with ointments and special shampoos and scalp lotions.

Neurodermatitis: This generally affects the base of the scalp and shows up as a clearly defined band of heavy scales with a sharp demarcation line between the affected patch and the adjacent normal healthy skin. It is probably one of the most horribly itchy of scalp disorders; scratching perpetuates the agony by stimulating the skin to produce a build-up of ever greater quantities of protective scales which harden while the skin beneath becomes red and tender. It is more common in post-menopausal women and seems to be linked with disorders of the central nervous system.

Problems associated with Hair loss

That the hair, along with the skin, should so accurately measure physical and emotional ups and downs is hardly surprising since hair cells, nourished by a constant supply of nutrients transported via the blood supply to the scalp tissues, reproduce themselves more rapidly than any other part of the body with the exception of bone marrow and liver tissue. For sheer intricacy and biological precision, the cycles and patterns of hair growth are hard to beat. On average, hair grows about 0.4 mm a day, which works out at between $\frac{1}{2}$ to $\frac{3}{4}$ of an inch a month. Each hair goes through three stages of development: anagen (the growing phase), catagen (the transition phase), and telogen (the resting phase), at which final point its own predetermined in-built lifespan prevents it from growing any further after it has reached a certain length, allowing it to fall out. Luckily, of course, these cycles are rarely synchronised, otherwise baldness would be commonplace! It *is* perfectly normal, however, to lose about thirty to one hundred hairs a day, although such loss rarely yields dramatic results since new growth is constantly underway. Subject to its own state of flux, growth too is governed by definite seasonal cycles, growing faster in summer than in winter — the traditional resting phase — and tending to grow in cycles of two and five years. Sudden, excessive or unduly prolonged hair loss or unusual thinning may prove an indication that the cycles have slipped slightly out of gear, shifting to a premature and perfectly normal resting phase. However, there could also be more insidious and menacing catalysts afoot, since hair growth can fall foul of a range of different stresses and stimuli which affect the circulation and ultimately the nourishment of scalp tissues, or alter the function of the central nervous system, hormone secretions and general metabolism.

Because it invariably exerts a vice-like grip on shoulder, neck and head muscles, nervous tension, for instance, contracts the arrector pili muscles that lie within the follicles themselves and restricts the flow of blood to the scalp, and so apart from creating headaches, it can also affect the growth of hair. Gentle head and neck massage and exercises to relax tense muscles also boost circulation and help to reverse the problem. Any sudden drop in hormone levels such as immediately after pregnancy or after stopping the Pill is a prime though temporary cause of hair loss. Contraceptive pills of the progestogen only variety or those with a fairly high progestogen content can, by depressing oestrogen production and causing other subtle biochemical changes in the body, precipitate excessive hair loss. Any over or under-activity of the thyroid gland, apart from wreaking other forms of physical havoc, is also recognised as a prime factor in thinning or falling hair — indeed falling hair is sometimes the *only* symptom of a low thyroid. Powerful drugs such as cortisone and more significantly the chemo-therapy and radiation used in the treatment of cancer are well-recognised as directly responsible for causing very severe hair fall or total baldness. Thankfully the baldness induced by chemo-therapy which kills off hair cells is invariably temporary, and when treatment has finished the hair grows back, normally within a few months. 'Mechanical' or self-inflicted damage can often show up as thinning or bald patches. The culprit usually turns out to be localised trauma or traction, such as wearing the hair very tightly gripped in curlers or in a pony tail and so exerting undue tension on the scalp tissues and hair follicles, massaging and rubbing of the front of the scalp which encourages hair to recede, and nervous picking and pulling of sections of hair which eventually causes patchy thinning. However, compared to such easily treatable temporary and often partial 'moulting' problems, none looms as large as the spectre of alopecia (the technical name for baldness), which includes so-called male pattern baldness, a phenomenon which because of its hormonal origin is not necessarily always confined only to men.

Androgen-dependent Alopecia

It was Aristotle who with characteristic prescience originally observed that the only way to prevent men from going bald was by castration. Simplistic as it sounds, the adage encapsulates the tyranny of man's — and woman's — hormonal system and makes the so-called paradox of baldness very easy to understand. Quite simply, the single cause of male pattern baldness as well as of androgen-dependent alopecia in women is a genetic sensitivity to androgens — the male sex hormones — which are produced in very large quantities in the testes, and in far smaller quantities in the ovaries and adrenal glands of women. Testosterone, which is the dominant catalyst in the development of baldness, acne and hirsuteness, circulates throughout the body via the bloodstream and eventually a small percentage of the hormone, roughly 1 to 2 per cent, is converted by special enzymes in the skin into a powerful by-product called dihydrotestosterone (DHT). And it is at this point that the trouble sets in. Depending on an individual's genetic blueprint, once DHT is synthesised, it may in certain individuals head straight for specific 'target cells' located principally in the hair follicles and oil glands, where it can cause acne in both sexes, hirsuteness in women, and baldness, through shrinking of the hair follicles, mainly in men, though also sometimes in women. It is the very same hormone and the very same idiosyncratic process responsible for adolescent pustules, boils, cysts and pimples, that triggers thinning of the temples and crown in a man of twenty-eight or thirty-five or embarrassing surplus body hair in a girl of eighteen. What's more, in adult women with an in-built genetic sensitivity to testosterone, any increase in male hormone levels and a decrease in oestrogen can set the scene for baldness which, though not as commonplace or well-recognised as male baldness, is inevitably more psychologically devastating and aesthetically and socially unacceptable.

Luckily endocrinology (the study of the hormonal system) and the study of genetics have advanced in leaps and bounds in recent years and therefore the logistics of testosterone and DHT production are now more fully understood, while radio-immunoassay and other techniques used to measure hormone levels in the blood and tissues have of late become incredibly refined. Normally testosterone is bound up with androgen binding globulin (ABG), a special protein manufactured in the liver, which renders it inactive and prevents it from homing in on those destructive target cells located in the skin. But in certain individuals the amounts of what's known as 'free' circulating androgens is higher than normal, possibly because of a deficiency in ABG, while in those people 'programmed' to go bald, the effect that this 'free' circulating hormone has when it latches on to the androgen receptors in the scalp or skin is to shrink the follicles. The reason why men lose their hair in an especially circumscribed manner and pattern is because only those parts of the scalp tissue that are genetically 'marked' as androgen-sensitive, in particular the crown and temples and hair line, are programmed to lose hair. In men the age at which the target cells begin to clamp down on hair growth varies tremendously. A man can begin to go bald in his early to mid-twenties and lose all his hair before the age of thirty. Male baldness is a subject still bedevilled by centuries of hand-me-down myths and cherished misconceptions. For every woman pursuing the chimera of everlasting youth in the cosmetics department, there exists a male desperado similarly stalking the trichology and hair care counters in a last bid to defy the laws of nature. And yet hair-loss *cannot* be arrested through external treatments such as massage, electrical stimulus, or the use of exotic herbal or organic scalp tonics to stimulate scalp tissues or hair. This is because male pattern baldness has nothing whatever to do with faulty circulation, tension, stress, or diet. It is a complaint which, according to all current scientific evidence, is caused by a genetically predetermined sensitivity to male sex hormones. It is amazing how many men who *are* aware of the hormonal link will use it as a syllogism in an attempt to bolster vanity and ego. But just because baldness is symptomatic of a man's reaction to his own androgens, and because eunuchs do not lose their hair, this does *not* automatically mean a bald man is more virile or has a greater sex drive than a man with a full head of hair! Studies show that baldness is not necessarily caused by excess amounts of androgens floating around in the system, but rather by its conversion into DHT and the geographic distribution of those follicles which are sensitive to that particular androgen.

In women, androgen-dependent alopecia begins far later in life, often not until the menopause, and its effects are not as pronouced or its progress as rapid. What is more, according to leading trichologist Philip Kingsley, baldness in women is curable provided treatment is prescribed soon enough. There does seem to be a point of no return in certain forms of hormone-linked hair loss, and if allowed to go untreated for too long it will reach a state where it is irreversible. There are diverse strategies for coping with hormones when they backfire, though for obvious reasons controlling the production of testosterone is far easier and less fraught with side-effects in women than in men! Assessing which androgens are produced in excess and evaluating which glands — ovaries or adrenals — are predominantly responsible for the over-production can help determine an effective mode of control. Oestrogen therapy helps to suppress androgens manufactured by the ovaries, while small amounts of corticosteroids can control androgens produced within the adrenal glands. If the liver is not manufacturing sufficient quantities of ABG to limit the amount of 'free' circulating androgens in the blood, then production of the protein can be stepped up with oestrogen or thyroid extract. Studies show that progesterone applied topically can reduce the formation of DHT in both men and women within the skin tissue, but dosage must be carefully monitored because in women the menstrual cycle can become disrupted if the concentration is too high. In certain cases supplementary zinc therapy can inhibit the enzyme that turns testosterone into DHT. Anti-androgen substances such as cyproterone acetate, used also to treat acne in women, reduce the levels of testosterone in the body, and when applied to the skin they block the skin's receptor sites, preventing conversion into DHT. However, systemic anti-androgens cannot be given to men, since the principal side-effects are lowered libido or impotence and sterility. Some dermatologists report good results in controlling male as well as female baldness with topical anti-androgen products, though as yet there is inconclusive evidence to support these claims. Research is currently underway to test the effectiveness of a group of anti-androgen substances which, instead of depressing the normal levels of testosterone in the bloodstream, instead block its conversion into DHT within the skin. By only inhibiting the activity of the hormone at the crucial target site — the skin itself — scientists hope that male as well as female baldness can be controlled without any of the side-effects of other anti-androgens. However such drugs are still very much in the early developmental stage, and until a breakthrough occurs, for male baldness at any rate, wearing toupées, hair weaves, or embarking on such costly, dubious, and often hit-and-miss cosmetic techniques as punch grafting (hair transplants) remains the only option to a thinning receding hairline and partial or total baldness. Not that punch grafting — taking small plugs of hair and tissue from those parts of the head still covered in hair and transplanting them into the bald parts — cannot sometimes do a good cover-up job. It can — and sometimes even quite realistically. However, there are only a handful of surgeons around the world who are truly adept at the skills needed for transplant work. The success of a transplant operation — which is usually carried out in two or three separate operations — depends on the characteristics of a man's hair-growth and how he normally wears and styles his hair, the way the donor grafts settle in and match up to the recipient site, and whether grafts are being used merely to fill in sparse areas of remaining hair or to fill up a totally denuded expanse of scalp. 'Returfing' a partly balding scalp is nowhere as easy or straight-forward as returfing a lawn that's past its prime. For every man proudly sporting a newly transplanted growth of hair, dense and naturally well-integrated, there are sadly a greater number of transplant failures whose grafts have failed to 'take' at all (a good example of this is the singer Elton John), whose scalps are scarred and dotted ugly-duckling style here and there with ragged tufts and wisps of straggly down, or others whose rigidly vertical plugs of hair have been deftly punched into parallel lines with all the precise symmetry of a neatly sown field of corn, thus giving the game away entirely.

Eyes

The eye area has a perverse tendency to add on years to a person's true age, even though the rest of the face remains smooth and unlined. The skin around the eyes is extra fine with very little fatty underlay or sebaceous glands. It is therefore likely to become dehydrated and develop lines, wrinkles, crêpiness, and creases before any other part of the face. Fatigue, hay fever, sinus problems, catarrh — which congests the tissues and make them swell up — crying, and using a set of highly animated facial expressions that involve crinkling and screwing up the eyes, further adds to the toll. 'Under eye bags' or puffiness can be hereditary or caused by using over-rich face creams and oils, and when the swelling becomes chronic and truly ageing, cosmetic surgery is the only sure-fire means of tightening and rejuvenating the lower lids. The body tends to retain fluid while asleep, and facial puffiness especially around the eyes is a common problem that can cause many men and women to look tired and groggy even after a good night's sleep. Puffy eyelids caused by excessive fluid retention can be controlled to a certain degree by avoiding the use of rich or heavy creams around the eyes, which can seep into the corner of the eye during the night and congest the tissues, and also by sleeping with the head somewhat elevated by several pillows, by a wedge under the head of the bed, or by propping up the box spring beneath your mattress by at least 4 inches. Ice-cold compresses — pads of cotton wool soaked in either cold tea or a strong solution of herbal Eyebright mixture — can help tremendously in reducing swollen eyelids during the day, while Clarins herbal based eye gel is second to none on the market in smoothing, tightening, and reducing swollen and congested tissues and ironing out small wrinkles and creases.

Contour changes where the lower eyelid meets the upper cheek area can also be caused by other factors. With ageing, a rift develops in the deeper dermal support tissues between the lower lid and the upper cheek. This 'separation' can eventually cause a broad, thin skinned, semi-circular depression to cleave itself into the tissue below the eye. This depressed area, especially if adjacent to fatty fullness near the lower lid, results in a deeply shadowed groove especially noticeable when lighting of the face comes from above. Some American cosmetic surgeons and dermatologists advocate the use of either silicone or collagen augmentation to fill in the groove that causes the shadow beneath the lower lid, but a far safer and effective alternative is to tackle the puffiness and swelling of the lower lid which is mainly responsible for causing the shadow in the first place. Dark circles under the eyes are certainly one of the most common cosmetic complaints which can appear even in the early twenties and generally intensify with time, and these can appear worse as a result of hyper-pigmentation of the skin of the lower eyelid and the upper cheek caused by excessive exposure to sunlight; eye glasses can aggravate the condition by focusing light on the lower lid and the upper cheek, and this intensified ultraviolet light exposure also makes the area a relatively common site of skin cancer in people who wear clear glasses in sunlight, which is why it is advisable to consult your eye specialist for special sunglass lenses to filter ultraviolet radiation. Other contributory factors to ageing and dark circles beneath the eyes are thinning of the surface skin which throws the blood supply network into greater relief and tints the skin a reddish-blue while also contributing to a greater visibility of tiny glands which are seen as small skin-coloured bumps, and the appearance of small brown spots, closed comedones (milia), and tiny broken veins. All these blemishes can be treated and eliminated successfully through either chemical exfoliation, electro-desiccation, cryosurgery, or dermabrasion.

Feet

The foot is a masterpiece of human engineering, brilliantly designed to support and balance the whole weight of the body in an infinite variety of positions and activities, and to act as a shock absorber and thus protect other limbs, joints and organs from injury. But by adapting perhaps too readily to strain and accommodating the pressures and distortions we inflict on our bodies through bad posture, over-activity, and the foibles of fashion, the foot, from a very early age, becomes the prime target of physical stress and imbalance. Nine out of ten people develop foot problems of one type or another before they reach their early twenties. Ill-fitting shoes and walking incorrectly, by creating excessive pressure and friction on parts of the foot, in turn lead to the formation of callouses, corns and more serious conditions such as enlarged toe joints and bunions. Regular scrubbing of the pressure edges around the ball of the foot, toes and heel with a pumice stone, and paring or clearing away the hard skin with a 'grater' or chiropodist's scalpel helps to avoid the callouses which form as a natural protective response to the effects of friction, pressure and body weight during walking. However, over-zealous removal of callous skin on the balls of the feet can expose very tender areas which may then develop blisters, so go easy when carrying out a home pedicure. Corns, which are simply a build-up of tough horny skin with a hard inner core that causes pain on nerve endings when you walk, respond best to early treatment from a chiropodist or a do-it-yourself corn removal plaster and/or liquid kit to soften keratin build-up so that the core can then be removed. Felt pads, plasters and 'buffer' sponges can minimise the pressure of shoes and protect heavy spots. Verrucas or plantar warts and athlete's foot are both highly contagious conditions which flourish in moist, dark, unhygienic surroundings and can be passed on by infected clothing, socks and towels. Verrucas usually need prompt professional attention to prevent them from growing more deeply and painfully into the tissues and multiplying. Athlete's foot, which some specialists believe may be caused by different species of fungi or bacteria, begins with rawness, itching, cracking or sogginess of the skin between the toes and may develop into scaling, blistering, and more widespread eruptions. To speed healing and prevent spreading, bathe frequently, dry the feet and between the toes thoroughly, use an anti-fungal powder, and apply a special athlete's foot tincture to clear up more serious infections. To further confuse the issue, athlete's foot is by no means the only cause of redness and rashes on the feet. Psoriasis, eczema and other allergic or irritant skin conditions can erupt to produce symptoms that are virtually identical to that of athlete's foot but do not respond to the usual treatment prescribed for this disorder. Proper nail care can help to prevent such painful disorders as ingrowing toe nails which are caused by narrow, ill-fitting shoes and also by cutting the nail too low at the corners, which allows the edge of the nail plate to dig into the soft tissue at the side. In very severe cases the area can go beyond redness and tenderness and become severely infected, and the nail plate or part of it may have to be removed. Toe nails should be cut in a straight line and then very gently filed to eliminate rough or jutting edges. Daily or twice daily bathing or showering followed by a foot refresher-cum-deodorant spray or foot powder helps to reduce a lot of the swelling, sweating, throbbing and other daily punishment meted out to feet that pound the city's pavements.

Hands

The condition and care of the cuticle, the opaque fold of skin at the base of the nail, greatly determines the way in which nails grow. It protects the nail fold from infection and must not be cut unless it is torn or ragged. Prodding, pushing or digging around the cuticle with sharp-edge or metal objects can cause indentation or ridges in the nail plate, yet the cuticle must be kept pliable and free of the nail otherwise it impedes growth and encourages surface irregularities and hang-nails which may become rough and cracked. A rich cuticle cream massaged into the nail and cuticle after bathing each night while pushing any protruding skin back gently with a rubber hoof stick should keep cuticles neat and soft. To avoid inflammation and tearing into the deeper living layers of the skin, hang-nails should be removed at the base with scissors as soon as they form.

It is easy to forget that nails nearly always bear testimony to physical health, although the evidence shows up belatedly since the average nail takes four to six months to grow out fully and the effects of illness will not show up until about three months after the illness first occurred. Taking certain medicines such as antibiotics or eating an unbalanced diet can, in the long-term, affect the strength and growth rate of nails. Wearing rubber gloves for household chores is the finest way of preventing dehydration of the skin on the backs of the hands and protecting the nails from the corrosive and weakening effects of detergents and other harsh chemicals. Wearing nail polish also helps to mitigate some of the effects of abrasive cleansers and chemicals on the nail including the problem of discoloration. Certain nail disorders are an extension of skin infections and should therefore be treated by a dermatologist. Onycholysis which includes crumbling, discoloration and separation of the nail plate from the nail bed, stems from a variety of dermatological disorders such as psoriasis, fungal infections including candida (thrush), an over-active thyroid, and as a reaction to certain drugs and externally applied chemicals. Formalin and chemical derivatives of for-maldehyde (present in most nail building and false nail kits) are particularly suspect, since all can trigger vicious allergic reactions such as dryness of the nail, bleeding, and discoloration discom-forts. Paronychia is the term used to describe swelling and inflammation of the soft tissue surrounding the nail plate. Due to anything from splinters and nail biting to keeping the hands immersed in water for long periods, the problem may become acutely aggravated through the formation of pus and abscesses which ultimately require draining.

Personal Hygiene

Excessive or profuse perspiration, especially if accompanied by an offensive odour triggered by the action of normal bacteria on the skin secretions, is undoubtedly one of the most embarrassing inflictions known to men and women alike. The problem is especially acute during adolescence and early adulthood when the oil as well as the sweat glands tend to be more active and their activity is boosted even further by nervousness, lack of self-confidence, and a nervous system generally hyped up by the pressures of exams, first jobs, and early romantic and sexual involvement with the opposite sex. For apart from physical exercise and heat, nervous tension is the prime trigger of sweat, whether produced by the apocrine glands situated mainly under the arms and in the groin, or the two to three million ecrine glands that lie scattered all over the face and body just beneath the skin surface. Ecrine sweat does not smell offensive but nevertheless it can prove uncomfortable and upsetting, especially when all around you are keeping their cool while you are losing it. Getting into a 'muck sweat' — damp palms, dewy upper lip, rivulets trickling down the spine making your clothes damp, moist sticky feet and soggy shoes — is as much a social problem as one connected with hygiene. Frequent bathing is of course the primary method of controlling body odour and perspiration, as is the regular use at least once a day of an effective aluminium chlorhydrate-based antiperspirant/deodorant product to neutralise odour by controlling the proliferation of underarm bacteria. No antiperspirant is able to control sweat secretion 100 per cent effectively — to do so the pores would have to be completely blocked off and excessive skin dryness would be the net result. As it is, certain extra-strong antiperspirants on the market which are designed to build up a perspiration barrier can all too easily cause an extreme irritant reaction and dry skin problems and rashes in many people.

Short of defusing emotional stresses, there is little — other than adhering to scrupulous and rigorous standards of hygiene, wearing loose-fitting clothes made from natural rather than synthetic fibres, and changing one's clothes daily — that can be done to eliminate the problem entirely. Sweating of the hands and feet can be treated by taking tablets containing atropine, which slows down the activity of the glands. However side-effects include upset stomach, a dry throat and mouth, and blurred vision. In cases of chronic underarm sweating, a portion of skin containing the largest concentration of glands beneath the arm can be removed or, alternatively, the nerve supply to the area can be severed. Cryosurgery — freezing the skin with liquid nitrogen — can also prove successful in certain cases. More recently a technique called iontophoresis has been developed which involves passing a special anti-sweating drug into the skin by charging it with a low-frequency galvanic current that facilitates osmosis. Treatment is painless, and as the sweat glands are plugged up, sweat production is drastically cut down for a period of weeks and months. Treatment can be given by a dermatologist if he has access to an iontophoresis unit, and it is commonly used to treat hands and feet.

CHAPTER 12

New for Old

Cosmetic surgery and allied rejuvenative treatments

Somewhere between the mid-thirties and the mid-forties we begin to accept, with as much good grace as vanity allows us to muster, the expression lines and quirky crinkles that represent the acceptable face of maturity. But once the crinkles turn to creases, the lines to folds, and the tracings deepen into etchings, acceptance may either develop into total resignation or increasingly into disgust or despair. Next follows the moment of truth when we realise that no matter how well we care for our skin or consult beauty therapists or take salon treatments, the *only* guaranteed method of appearing younger, and some would say more attractive, is cosmetic surgery.

Although thankfully we still rank far behind America in the neurotic and obsessive quest for physical perfection — eternal youth is America's holy grail, a pre-requisite for professional and social success — cosmetic surgery in Britain has, rightly, shed almost every vestige of stigma, all hint of taboo. Women are increasingly prepared to swap face-lift experiences and talk openly about their nose-jobs or eyelid tucks, while the number of men seeking corrective or rejuvenative surgery is, according to one leading British surgeon, growing steadily each year.

Complaints and dissatisfactions with regards to cosmetic surgery nearly always stem from the unrealistic demands and great expectations of women who expect a face-lift in particular to roll back the years along with the folds and wrinkles and return them to the unmarked perfection of their twenties and thirties. Yet the truth — unpalatable as it may be to many patients — is that cosmetic surgery provides no miracle cure against ageing. A face-lift cannot make a woman of fifty-five look twenty-five or even thirty-five. What's more, if you think about it, even if it could, the result would be grotesque. Of course a lot depends on at what stage in their life a person decides to opt for surgery. A woman who begins to undergo minor 'nips and tucks' such as tightening of the skin of the lower eyelids and a temporal face-lift (one that only tightens the upper half of the face) in, say, her late thirties, is in a sense using surgery as a preventive measure to minimise the approaching ravages of ageing, although the effects of surgery only last so long, say five to ten years maximum, and in order to maintain the same relative degree of youthful appearance at any given age, surgery must be repeated to keep up those deceptive appearances. There can be no firm rules regarding the 'right age' for surgery, and the criteria for surgery vary greatly. Often an otherwise smooth, firm, unlined face may *appear* older through puffiness and premature ageing of the eye area, hereditary pouches and swelling beneath the eye, lines of tiredness, deep crow's feet, and stretching and wrinkling of the fine skin, all of which create a demand for eyelid surgery. Loose, overhanging tissue on the upper lid can also give a 'closed eye' look at any age, causing a sleepy expression. Some women and men therefore may find that they need an 'eye-job' as early as their mid-thirties, while for older people eyelid surgery is often a necessary adjunct to a full face-lift.

But it's worth remembering that when those five or ten years are up, the people who have undergone surgery, whatever their age at the time, will still only look the same as they did *before* surgery; in other words, five or ten years younger than they probably otherwise would have looked without surgery. Early surgery, say in the forties or early fifties, rather than the late fifties, sixties, or even seventies, may prove less dramatic in the 'before' and 'after' sense, but it is therefore less likely to give the game away, for at best, although softening and greatly alleviating deep lines of tiredness and tension — vertical lines in particular — counteracting the downward pull of flesh and muscles as well as smoothing out the finer surface wrinkles and crêpiness in slack skin, surgery can make a man or woman look as if they have returned from a long relaxing holiday. Surgeons always stress that aiming for anything more ambitious or radical can lead to a taut, expressionless mask, overstretching the facial tissues, damage to the facial nerves, and distortion and discomfort — all in all a giveaway in every way!

'Beauty is a matter of a millimetre' is the way one leading

surgeon puts it, when it comes to designing a nose to fit a face, softly rounded breasts instead of aggressively rigid cones, and avoiding a set mask when redraping facial tissue and lifting sags and bags. The guiding maxim — better less than too much — is prevalent amongst the most successful and respected surgeons today. By playing safe, they leave room for further adjustments and avoid creating irreversible damage.

The Art of the Possible

There are other important provisos for successful surgery. Surgeons don't like to struggle over a salvage operation. American surgeons don't refer to cosmetic improvements as 'redraping' for nothing, since ideally any tightening manoeuvres and procedures for taking in the 'slack' should be performed before degenerative changes in the skin have gone too far. The best effects come from working with facial or body tissue that is still relatively springly or supple, and not too dehydrated or stippled with a cross-hatch of lines and grooves. Well-defined, strong, aesthetic bone structure is what finally determines the success of a face-lift whereby large areas of slack tissue have been tightened. Nor will a good surgeon operate on anyone who is more than a few pounds over-weight — patients must be as near as possible to their normal weight for any face or body operation to be successful. Times of emotional trauma, shock, illness, and bereavement are also no-go situations that may temporarily preclude surgery. Apart from advising patients on the potential limits of cosmetic surgery techniques — the art of the possible, and the impossible — tracing the real motivation behind any request for cosmetic surgery is one of the trickiest jobs of the specialist. Today's best surgeons are part-detective, part-psychiatrist, rooting out spurious psychological motives that could underpin the desire to look younger and more attractive. Too often, say top surgeons, minor physical imperfections become a convenient 'peg' on which to hang life's woes, be they professional, emotional or sexual. All to familiar is the role of 'Mr Feel-good/Fix-it' which is conferred on surgeons by potential patients with an obsessive and neurotic fear of becoming older, coupled with subconscious hopes that surgery will prove a life-transforming panacea for marital and emotional problems and loneliness. Would-be patients with such motives are strongly dissuaded from surgery. The motives surgeons most approve of? Honest vanity, the desire to look a bit younger, healthier, and more attractive as an end in itself. This is the most justifiable reason for surgery. Any reputable specialist will pull no punches: having a face-lift or eyes de-bagged, breasts recantilevered or firmed up, won't patch up a marital rift or cure depression.

Access

Having decided to undergo surgery, the task of finding a first-class reputable surgeon can prove daunting in the extreme, especially for those people who live outside central London or other big cities in Britain and have no one to pass on the names of top surgeons in this field. Silence and medical ethics continue to perpetuate the anonymity of Britain's top surgeons, a problem compounded by the fact that compared with their American peers, many British doctors still adopt a lingering puritan stance on the alleged trivial aspects of cosmetic surgery — an entrenched view that sternly condemns the folly of giving way to vanity at any age! And yet referral to a surgeon — as to any specialist —*must* come from a GP, and if he proves, as is too often the case, unsympathetic, patients may well find themselves caught in a medical impasse. Women whose looks may be the worse for weathering severe emotional stress or physical trauma are often advised to keep taking the valium and forget the wrinkles. Nature's 'wear and tear' remains, along with menopausal oestrogen-deficiency or pre-menstrual tension, women's biological heritage according to many conventional doctors all over the country, and the old adage still prevails — it's just your lot in life, and if it isn't life-threatening or painful, don't worry about it! Meanwhile victims of this Catch-22 situation have become an increasingly exploitable market for the unscrupulous, shady, 'cowboy clinics' run by medically unqualified businessmen, which have proliferated in recent years and which offer impartial advice on cosmetic problems and prompt arrangements for surgery. Alas, with one or two exceptions, the cosmetic surgery clinics that advertise freely in newspapers and magazines often lead patients not towards self-improvement but to mutilation. Consultation — not necessarily conducted by a doctor — is often perfunctory, arrangements may be made for clients to undergo surgery that they neither need nor in the interests of health and safety should undergo, the prices for surgical and clinic fees may be exorbitantly over-priced, and operations may be carried out by so-called leading surgeons who are not Fellows of the Royal College of Physicians (FRCP) or sometimes even accredited plastic surgeons. 'Horror stories' of surgeons who see their patients for the first time only in the operating theatre, botched-up operations, physical complications, cursory pre-operative consultations and post-operative care and maintenance, as well as general negligence, have become legend up and down the country, yet such unethical, unscrupulous organisations continue to flourish and will doubtlessly continue to do so for as long as doctors in general perpetuate the puritan ethic as far as aesthetic improvement is concerned.

Of course if your own GP *does* prove unsympathetic, you are fully within your rights to 'shop around' until you find a doctor who will refer you to a reputable cosmetic surgeon, a lengthy and often costly procedure, especially for anyone living outside a large town or city. If all else fails, you could ask your local hospital for the address of their nearest plastic surgery unit and the name of the surgeon in charge. He will generally see patients privately as well as on the NHS. If you really *are* compelled through circumstance to consult a clinic, find out the surgeon's name in advance and look him up in the Medical Directory at the local library to check whether he has the letters FRCS after his name or try to ascertain his credentials through the British Association of Plastic Surgeons. Whether you follow the ethical GP's referral or the private clinic route to cosmetic surgery, make sure you have a long and thorough consultation with the surgeon, discuss what it is you wish to have done, get him to tell you the possible pitfalls, and establish a rapport with him. His is a highly specialised field, as complex and liable to all sorts of trauma as many other forms of surgery, and added to this he needs the fine art of dealing with people's emotions, practising complex psychology regarding their looks, sex appeal, subjective ideas and aesthetics. After all, you have only one face and one body, and a single skin — all too precious to risk distortion, mutilation and permanent damage in the wrong hands. Cosmetic surgery is not something to be undertaken as lightly and with as little forethought as choosing a new hair-do or embarking upon a course of salon treatments. Some forms of surgery *can* prove painful (don't let anyone lull you into thinking that there is no pain ever involved in cosmetic surgery) depending upon the degree and area of improvement; mostly the aftermath of the operation merely involves discomfort, swelling, and bruising. Inevitably surgery will disrupt your lifestyle and schedule for some weeks, slowing you up and affecting your looks temporarily. Get the surgeon to explain what to expect, which will be different in each individual case, according to skin type, age, rate of healing, etc.

Eyes

Cosmetic surgery of the eyelids (blepharoplasty) is immensely popular, very safe, and extremely successful. It can take years off a man or woman's face, often postponing and even eliminating the need for a face-lift. It seems a paradox that while the delicacy of the tissues around the eyes make them the most prone to ageing, discoloration, thinning and wrinkling, and puffiness, it also makes them the most responsive to surgery. The skin heals very rapidly, leaves no scarring, and the results are generally long-lasting. An added bonus is that temporary swelling and marking can be camouflaged with eye make-up, so that there is little trauma or upheaval in the patient's lifestyle.

'Under eye bags' are caused generally by tiny nodules or so-called fatty hernias embedded in the flesh of the lower eyelid. Additional accumulation of fat and fluid can stretch the skin and weaken the underlying membrane that normally holds the tissues flat and in place, thus giving slack eye contours. Making a fine and tiny incision just beneath the rim of the lower lid, the surgeon can easily take out these fatty deposits, tighten the membrane and slack skin a fraction, and so iron out the whole area. Small lines are sometimes eliminated into the bargain, although true crow's feet, those deeper laughter lines that radiate out from the corner of the eye, cannot be effectively removed with this procedure unless the orbicularis muscle surrounding the eye from lid to socket is also tightened to smooth and minimise deep crow's feet, at present a procedure only undertaken by a few skilled surgeons in America. Crêpiness and small vertical lines and creases beneath the eye, which are more a product of skin degeneration than facial movement, can usually be tightened and ironed out through lower lid surgery. The main danger inherent in the removal of excess tissue around the eyes is that of ectropion — the lower lid flipping open and giving a 'blood-hound' look, as a ridge of fibrous tissue forms around the inner lid. Due to the sudden pulling away of too much skin, ectropion is ugly and uncomfortable, but in all except very rare and severe cases it is a temporary condition. It is more likely to occur if the patient has had more than one eyelid operation, and surgeons are disinclined to perform the operation twice as the skin on the eyelids can go slack.

Another danger involved in operating on the upper and lower lids is that, if too much skin is pulled back, it can cause a webbing effect at the outer corners of the eye. Performed by a reputable surgeon, the removal of eye bags should be free of complications. It involves about one week to ten days of swelling and bruising, and about one night in hospital unless the operation has been conducted on an out-patient basis. Many surgeons prefer the patients to be given a local rather than a general anaesthetic so that they can cooperate in keeping their eyes open and mobile which contributes very much to final aesthetic effects. In order to reconstruct a loose or overhanging upper lid, the incision is made in the natural fold of the skin and the excess flesh trimmed away. Recent refinements ensure that other hereditary defects can be reversed or corrected. In addition to removing surplus skin and fat on the upper lid, a section of the muscle can also be trimmed to open up the eye. Congenitally heavy lids or those with masking skin folds, such as in the oriental eye, are resculptured this way, so that the level at the upper lashline when the eye is open is adjusted. Putting the crease back in the eye at a slightly different level allows the surgeon to tailor the correct aesthetic proportions. The most important part of this operation is to gauge the exact proportions of the space between the rim of the upper lashes, the lid crease and the brow bone, so as to 'open up' the eye area and create a young expression. For this reason most surgeons prefer to carry out this operation also under a local anaesthetic so that the eyes remain open and the correct overall perspective of the eye area is maintained.

Another new development is the 'brow lift'. The angle of the eyebrows can contribute an ageing effect, giving a depressed, tired or scowling expression. The point of fixation of the eyebrows is freed from the underlying bone, allowing the surgeon selectively to adjust the shape of the brows. Says one London surgeon: 'It's the same process of snipping muscles that hold the frown line in place. We loosen the muscles which fix the brows and adjust them to give a more pleasing expression. The combination of frown lines and heavy brows can be one of the most ageing characteristics of a face.' The cost of tightening the lower lids is about £600, upper and lower lids £900.

Face-lifts

Cosmetic surgery is too costly and too drastic a step to allow for trial and error, and it's important to ascertain the limits as well as the possibilities of a face-lift. Degenerative changes that can most definitely be reversed or corrected through surgery are loose cheek tissues, deep nose to mouth folds and lines, a slack flabby chin and jowls, and some sections of wrinkled skin around the eyes. The success of a face-lift is based largely on the laws of cause and effect. Essentially it entails redraping whole areas of flabby and slack flesh on the face. The techniques of this type of surgery ensure that contours and curves are firmed and lifted, yet certain wrinkles and lines that are not an intrinsic extension of these contours may never be entirely removed. Therefore wrinkles that are caused mainly by loss of elasticity and moisture within the epidermis have little to do with slack muscles and flabby connective tissue and more with the overall condition of your skin. This is why on a long-term basis a face-lift is no substitute for early and preventive skin care. A surgeon can excise surplus fat; he cannot put collagen and moisture back into your skin, and the marks of age that are less easy to eliminate through surgery are small vertical lip lines, vertical frown lines, and horizontal tram-lines across the forehead. But the combination of worry lines and depressed, scowling eyebrows can be one of the most ageing aspects of the face, and by snipping and loosening the tiny muscles that fix the eyebrow close to the underlying bone, heavy brows can be lifted along the frown line to give a smoother, more relaxed and younger expression. The forehead can be tightened and smoothed to a certain extent by making a careful incision along the hairline and pulling up enough surplus flesh to alleviate the lines without making the area immobile. In addition to this procedure, some surgeons loosen or cut away part of the tiny corrugator muscles between the eyebrows that hold a vertical frown line in place through tension. By freeing the frontalis muscle along the centre of the forehead which elevates the brows, stubborn horizontal lines and furrows can usually be removed.

In a standard face-lift, the incisions are made partly in front of the ear within the natural crease and curved neatly behind the ear. Other incisions lie hidden right up within the hairline. There should be no scars whatsoever in the area between the back of ear and the hairline itself. Surgeons today expect a woman who has had a face-lift to be able to wear even very cropped or severely swept-up hair styles with absolute impunity. During the operation, which always entails a general anaesthetic, surplus skin and flesh are peeled back in a process called 'undermining'. The surplus is removed and the skin is tightened, redraped and stitched back snugly at an upward angle. Modifications to this basic method are few. However some leading American and British surgeons have now perfected a means of undermining, removing and manipulating not just skin but bands of flesh and muscle such as the platysma which run along the neck and up to the face. These muscles can be redraped to firm a flabby chin and loose neck tissues, resculpt a weak or poorly defined jaw, and mould a hereditary straight neck lacking contour — defects not necessarily connected with ageing. Loose neck muscles are partially excised or cut, sutured (sewn) together under the chin, and orientated in a different direction — usually swinging back to the sides of the jaw to form a sling or hammock. Removal of fatty tissue is also more radical today: to lift the neck and lower face the surgeon may de-fat the entire chin area, taking out a horseshoe-shaped crescent of fat around the jaw. Surgeons admit that this involves working very close to the nerves, and since there is the possibility of a greater incidence of nerve problems the operation requires more skill than simpler lifting procedures. Recontouring the lower face can be complemented by inserting a silastic chin implant for added definition. Muscle surgery may continue with modification of the cheek muscles — often necessary for older faces or in cases where advanced skin and connective tissue degeneration has started, and where the underlying bone structure is insufficiently prominent to give a good effect once the skin has been tightened. One surgeon uses the bizarre analogy of tightening 'perished rubber sheeting' when merely tightening loose skin to smooth the face.

Advanced surgery modifies the superficial musculo apeneurotic system, SMAS, which includes the extension of the platysma muscle and constitutes a tough fascia layer above the nerves. The SMAS layer is undermined, lifted, and a portion removed depending on the amount of laxity in the system. This allows tightening of the connective tissue and muscles which greatly helps the lifting of the cheeks, the nose to mouth fold, and relaxed jowls. The skin is then redraped over the tissue, giving a more natural contour. Surgeons say that as the skin isn't pulled over bulging tissues, this avoids any tension and the risk of a set mask look. Paradoxically, bruising and swelling are decreased as the skin avoids traumatisation, and scars heal more quickly and to a higher quality due to a lack of tension. Recovery rate is also the same as in standard surgery, although muscular procedures can extend the operation by twenty or thirty minutes. A stay in hospital is generally no longer than two or three nights and bandages are usually removed after twenty-four hours. There is often considerable swelling of the face, haematoma (bleeding beneath the skin) and bruising, depending on basic skin and body type, which subsides over a period of between five days and three weeks depending on the individual. Light make-up can generally be worn about five days after the operation when the stitches have been removed. Electromagnetic or pulsed high-frequency therapy applied immediately after the operation helps to decongest the tissues, calm down irritation, eliminate swelling, and generally promote quick and efficient healing and avoid the risk of scarring. It also greatly reduces the risk of infection. Treatment with creams and serums can help to improve the newly redraped skin surface and allow it to settle more quickly. It is obvious that revised make-up techniques and products are also an essential part of complementing a face that's younger, firmer and healthier. The cost of a full face-lift is between £1500 and £2000.

When feeling and looking our most tired, a lot of us have surely experimented with instant rejuvenation. Look in the mirror and gently pull back the skin on the temples. The result? You look less glum and fraught, crow's feet diminish, under eye circles and slackness are ironed out, and the face generally looks rested and younger, less pinched and tired. It was precisely in order to take in any minor 'slack' in a relatively young face that the 'mini-lift' was created — and why it proved so popular during the 1960s and 1970s. The operation, often performed under a local anaesthetic on an outpatient basis, involves making small diagonal incisions in the hairline above the temples and just pulling back the skin to iron out minor lines and wrinkles. There is no undermining and no fat is removed. Its effects therefore are limited to the area around the eyes and to a lesser extent light nose to mouth folds. The greatest drawback is the brevity of the rejuvenation period. Nips and tucks only last until gravity and facial stress pull them down again, so by its very nature the mini-lift has a limited life span. Today many surgeons, wise after the event, emphasise that there is little actual repair work that a mini-lift can achieve which cannot be avoided in the first place by weight control, good health, assiduous skin care, and possibly under eye surgery to tighten bags and slack tissue. If slackness, wrinkles, and ageing of the upper part of the face are a problem, surgeons may suggest that a man or a woman undergoes a temporal face-lift which involves only making incisions in the temple and possibly around the upper ear and only undermining and redraping the facial tissues of that part of the face.

Dermatological Patchwork

Rejuvenation is by its nature relative and therefore a fickle business. Sometimes a face-lift may be insufficient to improve greatly the skin and facial kept contours; sometimes on the other hand it is altogether uncalled for. Since the success of a face-lift depends to a large degree on where you show signs of wear and tear, 'facial geography' has a lot to do with defining the art of the surgically possible. Certain lines and wrinkles simply do not respond much to surgery no matter how deft the scalpel work: these include the vertical lines and furrows that cut down into the upper lip and fuzz up the lip line, crow's feet or misnamed 'laughter lines' and certain grooves and dents that cause shadows beneath the eye, and any network of wrinkles that traverses the forehead and cheeks at right angles or diagonally to the main facial curves. In addition to radical cosmetic surgery, however, there is a choice of dermatological back-up which surgeons use increasingly in order to obtain their finest rejuvenative effects. Techniques such as dermabrasion, chemical peeling, collagen injections and very occasionally silicone injections, cryosurgery and electro-desiccation belong to this modern crop of high tech cosmetic aids. These are often important surgical adjuncts, and while they require virtually as much skill as plastic surgery they nevertheless qualify as parasurgery, often conducted on an out-patient basis and used either on their own or to complement face-lifting techniques.

Resurfacing

Dermabrasion and chemical peeling or chemo-surgery are today widely accepted forms of therapy for many skin complaints and are used with a particularly high success rate to alleviate and minimise surface lines and wrinkles. Sadly there is a high failure rate in the treatment of severe acne or ice-pick scars — a condition most frequently referred to peeling or dermabrasion therapy. Although superficial acne scars, abnormal pigmentation, freckles and skin damage from UV radiation do respond well to chemical peeling, deep scars will often appear more pronounced against the fresh new skin. Large pores may also appear larger after peeling, and features such as moles and dilated blood vessels sometimes show up more. Chemo-surgery and dermabrasion are both highly effective for gaining a 'new' complexion, but both procedures involve an intense but short-term amount of discomfort and unsightliness.

Peeling is induced by painting a caustic phenol or other caustic solution onto parts of or the entire area of the face. A mask is applied and tightly taped onto the skin and worn for forty-eight hours. This is then removed, peeling off the burnt skin to expose the newly formed tissue underneath. The result is far from a pretty picture: symptoms over a one-week period or sometimes longer are similar to those of a severe second-degree burn — pain, weeping, swelling, reddening, the formation of a crust which must be kept soft by the regular application of ointments. After this follows a period when the face is very red, and as this diminishes the new skin is formed. Make-up can be used about seventeen days after the treatment and a sunscreen must be worn, although it is preferable to remain out of the sunlight altogether for a few months after a chemical peeling. In some cases the new skin may be blotchy and a second peel can take place after three or four months on the pigmented areas. Due to the fact that chemo-surgery induces a permanent reduction of the melanin producing cells in the basal layer of the epidermis, the skin may in some cases fail to repond normally to the sun and the patient will not be able to develop an even sun tan. A strong sunscreen must always be used — blotching on a new skin is invariably due to indiscriminate exposure to sunlight.

Dermabrasion, or skin planing, involves destroying the upper layers of the skin with a high-speed rotary disc or a carborundum brush attached to a high-speed drill. The skin is first anaesthetised and stiffened through freezing with jets of ice-cold 'liquid snow' such as ethyl chloride. Dermabrasion is most frequently used by doctors to treat acne marks and scars, and the removal of these pits and other defects can be precisely controlled both by choosing the correct width and diameter of wire brush and the correct degree of abrasiveness — the brushes are available in soft, regular and coarse grades. The selection of the appropriate abrasive instrument depends on the thickness of the skin and the depth of the scarring to be abraded. The speed of the motor driving the wire brush can be very precisely controlled, and the brush itself is moved by the surgeon over the frozen skin with a firm and steady back and forth motion with greater pressure applied to areas of deeper scarring. This is also an excellent treatment for such defects as stubborn lines and wrinkles, and patchy irregular areas of hyper-pigmentation. As with chemical peeling, however, the skin takes two or three weeks to heal, an often uncomfortable and unsightly process. During this period it is vitally important to have the dressings changed regularly and to take a course of antibiotics to prevent infection, and oral corticosteroid to reduce inflammation and oedema; antibiotic creams and ointments must also be applied in the post-operative period to speed healing, prevent infection, and keep the skin and the newly formed crusts soft. The new tissues remain pink or red for several weeks, and normal skin tone returns gradually in two to three months. During this time you can wear make-up but not go into the sun. It's worth remembering that while you are acquiring a new skin this can sometimes be at the cost of pigment cell destruction within the deeper epidermal cells. It may well be difficult to cultivate an even suntan after dermabrasion, and you'll need to make sure that you wear a strong and effective sunscreen whenever you expose your face to the sun. Men can resume shaving about ten days after the operation.

Restoration

Make no mistake, whatever beauticians may claim to the contrary, neither chemical peeling nor dermabrasion are fast healing, painless, full-proof short cuts to a new complexion. Nor can results always be guaranteed, since the even formation of healthy new skin depends very much on individual skin type and colouring in particular. The fairer the skin the better the results will be; the darker the complexion the higher the risk of blotchy pigmentation, and doctors are notoriously loath to perform a peel or dermabrasion on coloured skins or even on people with brown eyes, since there is always the danger of ending up with a bleached, slightly mottled effect.

Smaller and less pronouced skin imperfections such as individual brown spots, acne scars, tiny spider veins, actinic keratoses (dark, wartlike, non-cancerous growths caused by sun exposure) can be simply and rapidly eliminated by either cryosurgery or electro-desiccation, both carried out by dermatologists or in some cases by cosmetic surgeons within minutes on an out-patient basis. Cryosurgery or 'freeze therapy' consists of literally freezing the cells that present the problem, which causes them then to flake and peel off. Short sharp bursts of ethyl chloride, solid sticks of CO_2 (dry ice) or liquid nitrogen are most frequently used to freeze areas of hyper-pigmentation or raised non-cancerous bumps and lumps. After treatment the skin becomes red and blistery, then eventually turns brown and peels off like a bad sunburn. In certain cases cryosurgery may be used to kill skin cancer cells. It is also increasingly used for acne patients to improve localised pitting when dermabrasion would be too extreme a treatment. Where pinpoint precision is needed, in particular to remove broken blood vessels, spider nevae, sun spots, tiny enlarged glands, even freckles, electro-desiccation, whereby an electric current is applied via a very fine electric needle to burn away the pigmented or blemished area, may prove a viable alternative. The treated area turns red and forms a scab which, after a week or so, peels off, revealing the new unblemished skin beneath. However fast and painless these methods, it is worth remembering that both cryosurgery and electro-desiccation do slightly 'rough up' the epidermis and it takes about two weeks for the skin's appearance to return to normal.

Silicone and Collagen implants

Euphemisms abound in the beauty business but none are quite as irritating as the term 'expression lines', used to describe the creases and furrows we develop from the way we use our faces. Yet it is true that the formation of certain characteristics such as crow's feet (laugh lines but no laughing matter!) and tram-lines (frown or worry lines) often have little to do with age but are an index to the vocabulary of sadness, happiness, concentration, and the myriad other emotions that give the human face its individual identity. Perhaps this illustrates the saying that after a certain age we're stuck with the face we deserve. But are we? Although surgical face-lifts are only suitable for an older face, filling in the lines and furrows that mar an otherwise youthful face or an older one that proves stubbornly resistant to surgical redraping is something dermatologists in America have been trying to perfect for the last few years with varying degrees of success. The pros and cons of silicone versus collagen injections or implants are a thought-provoking, pivotal issue in today's treatment of ageing skin and make up a controversy that continues to rumble throughout medical circles. The points are well worth pondering, even though collagen *is* more widely available these days especially in Britain than silicone, for which you would have to do some pretty nifty shopping around.

It's worth remembering that all the brouhaha and scare stories regarding silicone go back to the 1950s and 60s when impure industrial-grade silicone was injected by unethical surgeons straight into the tissues, usually to augment the breasts. The result of this treatment was indeed horrific, with recorded cases of infection, leakage, cancer, the migration of silicone to other parts of the body — and even death. The type of silicone used today by only a handful of specially licensed surgeons in America (the American FDA has not passed the substance for cosmetic use) is, in contrast, highly-refined, pure, medical-grade silicone, which has been used successfully on thousands of people in very minute quantities to plump out facial lines, deep scars and wrinkles. Only a few tiny drops of silicone at a time are injected beneath the skin at well-spaced intervals. Injected properly — possibly over five sessions or more — silicone does not migrate to other parts of the body. On the contrary, a fibrous network of tissue forms around the substance, suspending it and holding it into place. If too much is injected, however, it may harden — and cannot then be removed. A more accessible, and to doctors and patients alike acceptable, method of skin rehabilitation, is collagen injections, which are used in much the same way and for the same skin problems as liquid silicone and are now widely available in America, Britain, and the rest of Europe. Though its long-term effects and lasting power remain to be seen, collagen certainly so far appears to be the safest method, both for people who do not yet need or want to undergo surgery and those for whom face-lifting has not fully removed certain stubborn lines and wrinkles. Implants are based on fine lightweight animal collagen (taken from cattle), which closely resembles that of human skin and is used in a way that can be compared to the irrigation of a dried-out river bed. The collagen is incorporated into a 70 per cent carrier fluid — a harmless saline solution plus a dash of lidocaine to act as a local anaesthetic — and injected within the skin layers in one fine liquid 'thread' along the line or wrinkle. Unlike silicone, which is placed beneath the skin surface (subdermally), collagen is injected within the skin layers (intradermally) to achieve the desired effects. In order to obtain a successful result an excess amount of fluid must be injected, often at various levels of the connective tissue, temporarily swelling the skin surface. However, this effect disappears in a couple of hours as the carrier solution dissipates, leaving only a residual 'bed' of collagen to be incorporated into the connective tissue which clings around it, holding it in place and filling out the indentation or 'trough' that is made by the wrinkle.

Because the body recognises collagen as a 'friendly' substance — it is after all the principal component of connective tissue — a network of blood vessels and new tissue cells are rapidly sent out to surround and colonise the implant which, after a few months, becomes indistinguishable from the normal host tissue. Some doctors are understandably cautious about the possible risk of an allergic reaction to collagen (although in America allergic reactions have occurred in only ten cases out of over three thousand), and those surgeons who use the American product Zyderm insist that each patient first undergoes a test shot followed by a four-week waiting period. Areas that respond best of all to collagen implants are vertical lip creases, frown furrows, horizontal forehead lines, vertical nose to mouth or cheek laugh lines, and certain scars including those that have arisen as a result of skin grafting, all areas notoriously hard to improve even with a face-lift. Depending on the depth of the facial lines, two or three injections may be needed before they are filled out, and the effects last from six months to a year, and often longer, depending on individual facial characteristics, after which time the collagen implant may require topping up. Unlike silicone, collagen cannot drift or harden in the body, but on the debit side neither does it have silicone's staying power. Which means that at around £100 for a single implant (or a twin 'set' of implants, as in the case of nose to mouth lines) on-going yearly collagen injections can prove a costly exercise in rehabilitation. Many American dermatologists and surgeons disagree on the merits of collagen, especially when compared to silicone; the main caveat — now that Zyderm has gone through a three-to-four-year term of trial and extensive cosmetic use — is that its effects fall far short of sensational, let alone guaranteed, especially on anyone who has deeply etched lines or wrinkles. What with the frequent inability of Zyderm fully to plump up lines for any long period of time, coupled with its acknowledged rate and degree of resorption, the ends, say many specialists, may simply not justify the cost. What is more, there are areas and problems in which Zyderm is ineffective. These are very deep acne or 'ice-pick' scars (better faded by being punched out and then sutured back together or filled with silicone), chicken-pox marks, and small superficial skin creases like those underneath the eye which are caused by excess and droopy skin. Nor can Zyderm — or silicone for that matter — be used to improve, correct, or fade existing stretch marks on any part of the body.

In 1983 a super double-strength collagen solution, Zyderm 2, was introduced on to the American market and is being used by a handful of British specialists. Consisting of 65 per cent collagen in a saline suspension, as opposed to 30 per cent collagen in the original formula, doctors are optimistic that this heavier-duty formula could well give silicone a run for its money — it will need to, because Zyderm 2 injections cost twice as much as regular Zyderm. Some specialists foresee that Zyderm 2 may score where Zyderm 1 has so far failed to deliver the goods: in filling up deeper scars, even those caused by acne, and in treating deeper lines and wrinkles, although it has been agreed even by the manufacturers of Zyderm, that in order to gain full benefits, skin should basically be young and in good condition, smooth rather than coarse, normal and oily rather than very dry. People in their fifties and sixties, whose skin has already lost its elasticity and undergone degenerative changes, usually fail to show any significant improvement as a result of collagen injections.

The Body

The Breasts (Augmentation)

Risks such as extensive and permanent scarring, loss of sensitivity, unnatural looking contours, the formation of hard inner scar tissue, infection, and other horrors are thankfully very rare nowadays, provided the operation to increase the volume of small breasts or fill out those that are sagging is undertaken by a surgeon who is experienced and up on all the latest techniques and choice of implants. For breast augmentation has in the 1980s reached a zenith of perfection. Incisions are usually tiny, made within the natural fold beneath the breast or, more ingeniously still, implants are inserted via tiny horizontal incisions in the armpit, eliminating giveaway marks altogether. There is no reason for augmented breasts not to look and feel 100 per cent natural, for today's implants or prostheses are masterpieces of brilliant deception, having the weight and feel of human tissue. Implants are breast-shaped, squashy envelopes of clear plastic, filled with liquid silicone gel and a saline solution. Newest refinements include the double-pocketed implant — the inner one contains silicone, the outer one a saline solution which can be topped up or reduced in volume at any time after the operation via a tiny syringe. New, too, are prostheses which are divided into three segments or sacs so that less silicone is needed, and the liquid itself is lighter and doesn't flow around the inner sac; with this design the chances of distortion or hardening are far less than with the older models. Implants are placed against the chest wall beneath the tissues, which minimise any risk of their masking any lumps, bumps or cysts. Women who have had babies are able to breast feed normally if they have had the operation, and only in rare cases does scar tissue form around the implant causing the breasts to harden — in which case the prosthesis may have to be removed. Some doctors advocate that a woman should massage her breasts regularly for about six months after the operation to prevent the formation of scar tissue.

Post-mastectomy Augmentation

Over the past few years an increasing number of women are also undergoing reconstructive surgery following a mastectomy, since most doctors now believe that this does not increase the risk of recurrence of tumours nor inhibit future diagnosis or examination. Augmentation may take place at the same time as the mastectomy, but more usually follows six months after healing is complete. Conditions for post-mastectomy augmentation include negative histology reports on tissue taken from the area, cases where the type of cancer has a good prognosis, i.e. was confined to breast ducts and nipple, and early detection and surgery, where the cancer was detected in the first stage, was less than two centimetres in size, and there is no evidence that it has spread. Augmentation of course does not mean that a woman will gain perfect proportions. It is an evening-out process by which sometimes even the other breast may be made smaller. Many patients confess that having a mastectomy makes them feel defeminised, castrated, even maimed. Losing a breast is, understandably, just like losing a limb to many women. The main problem of this operation is that the remaining tissues in the area can sometimes be too burnt and damaged after surgery and/or radiation to allow undermining, therefore the augmentation may be in two stages. Stage one repairs the damaged tissue using a flap transfer method of muscle and overlying skin from the back to the side of the rib cage. This is called the latissimus-dorsi-myocutaneous flap, which pivots healthy skin and muscle from the back to the front of the chest wall providing both the support and covering for a breast reconstruction. It leaves a six-inch scar on the back which, however, is usually covered by a brassiere. This operation also has the added advantage of introducing a fresh supply of blood to the area. If the original nipple is intact, it is sent for histology to ensure that it is free of carcinoma, and then saved for future use in completing the new breast. However a new nipple can be made by taking tissue from other parts of the body. Provided the medical history is well analysed and the area is free from possible carcinoma, there is no reason why a woman cannot have her breasts evened-out. Some even find the flap transfer sufficient, as it improves the damaged site.

Reduction

This presents much more of a major challenge to surgeons as it constitutes a major operation often fraught with pitfalls unless the volume and dimensions are calculated precisely to the last quarter of an inch. Removal of over-stretched excess skin and surplus tissue may involve considerable scarring, distorted shape and asymmetry of the breasts, and loss of sensation in the nipple. Incisions may be made vertically on the lower curve of the breast and round the areola, and sometimes along the fold under the breast. Excess skin, fat and tissue are removed, and the skin draped without tension to ensure fine scar lines. The nipple is usually lifted — though not completely detached — and re-positioned for an evenly balanced aesthetic effect. A certain loss of sensation, sometimes only temporary, may result after the operation, although by avoiding damage to the nerves a clever surgeon can greatly minimise the *degree* of sensitivity lost. If sagging is moderate to mild, an incision around the areola to pull up surrounding or underlying slack tissues may be all that's needed. In major body surgery such as breast reduction the amount and quality of scarring also depends very much on how skilled and nimble is the surgeon's stitchwork; extra care must be taken to avoid tension and pull on the newly draped tissues when incisions are joined. Specialised fine stitching techniques, sometimes using a Z formation to reduce tension, the use of fine adhesive paper tape, which by flattening the scar through constant pressure minimises the risk of bunching and hardening of scar tissue, and the use of staples to hold the tissue together in a neat line without tugging can create a world of difference between unsightly 'butcher's' marks and the discreet hallmark of a master surgeon. Younger women who undergo breast reduction should remember that there is no guarantee that they will be able to breast feed a child following surgery — the odds are about 50/50. Side-effects such as scarring and loss of sensitivity notwithstanding, many women are all too happy to trade these for such serious physical problems as the weight and pain of big breasts which may become agonising with added pre-menstrual volume, the ulceration caused by bra straps digging into the shoulder tissues, breasts sometimes so large that they become fluid-filled and can develop ulcers, and back pain caused by the sheer weight of the breasts.

Stomach
Abdominoplasty also constitutes major surgery but can give

excellent results, fading, ironing out or even eliminating stretch marks and old Caesarean or appendix scars, and tightening crêpy, wrinkled, loose skin which, no matter how much a woman diets or how assiduously she exercises or how tight and firm her tummy muscles, can and will never revert to its former resilience and smoothness, especially if she has had more than one or two pregnancies or lost a lot of weight. A horizontal incision is made above the pubis or bikini line and, leaving the navel intact, the flesh is pulled back to the ribs, the excess trimmed away — sometimes removing as much as half of the stomach skin — and the skin then pulled down 'like a snug vest' as one surgeon put it, leaving a fine almost imperceptible faint scar along the bikini line. The navel or umbilicus is brought through a new aperture, a scar running neatly around the edge. Recovery time can prove uncomfortable, with very definite limits on movement; two-days bed rest with knees bent is followed by ten to fourteen days when movement and walking is severely restricted to a crouching or semi-concave position. The upper inside 'thigh lift', successful on women with flabby sagging loose skin on the upper thighs, though inadvisable for anyone with thick heavy thighs, is carried out in an almost identical fashion — the bikini line scar is the same, although there may also be additional scars hidden away in the fold of the groin.

Arms

Recent additions to body sculpting and redraping include dermabrasion of the backs of the hands — often a giveaway after someone has lost years off their face and/or body — to eliminate patchy pigmentation, brown, blotched crêpiness, and roughness. After dermabrasion, the new skin that forms contracts automatically and exerts a tightening of the skin's surface. Very loose skin can also be pulled up, excised and tightened along the outside edge down to the little finger. Crêpey hanging skin around the elbows can be eliminated very neatly by cutting straight across beneath the bone — because it's a transverse and not a vertical incision, this is what surgeons refer to as a 'good scar' with little tension, fast and complete healing, fading, and no risk of keloid bunching. Less inconspicuous is the scarring involved in upper arm surgery (brachioplasty) for tightening loose, puckered skin and wobbly tissues between the armpit and elbow. The operation is easy enough to accomplish and the results are successful, but the scar which runs from the inner side of the elbow right up to the armpit cannot be hidden except by wearing long or three-quarter length sleeves.

Legs/Bottom

Operations to reduce the size of heavy or bulging upper thighs and large or 'dropped' buttocks seem simple enough theoretically and on paper — a crescent-shaped line is traced around the buttocks and hips to indicate where fatty tissue should be removed. But this is a major operation — blood loss, risk of complications and scarring can be extensive — and because more than any other this area of the body is subject to the downward pull of gravity, the final effect may prove asymmetrical and initial tightness, cantilevering and 'uplift' can, in a short period, droop and become pulled out of shape again. Moreover, post-operative recovery is usually slow and uncomfortable, requiring one week in hospital when the patient is generally unable to sit down or move about. Restriction on movement may last anything from two to four weeks.

But certain surgeons who might previously have had staunch objections to carrying out thigh or buttock reduction have been using a relatively new technique called suction curettage which was developed in France and is still the subject of tremendous controversy, mainly regarding both its immediate and long-term benefits. It is a bizarre-sounding operation, that hardly conjures up a pretty or appetising picture; excess fat is first liquified with injections of the enzyme hyaluronidase, mixed with a saline solution; the fat cells swell up and become very fragile, and then are literally siphoned off down a hoover-like tube into a jar! The suction cannula, as it's called, is inserted into the tissues, avoiding the blood vessels, through small incisions less than one inch long, made at two or three points on the thighs, hips or buttocks, and their position is strategically calculated to maintain the gently undulating convexity-concavity of the buttocks. Because fat is removed at 2 centimetres beneath the skin surface, doctors maintain that they are able to avoid surface dimpling or rippling, but reports filtering through from Europe indicate that considering the cost and discomfort involved results generally fall far short of expectations. Worse still than surface unevenness, some patients have complained of the formation of hard scar tissue and the eventual return of surplus fat. Fat cells once removed do not come back, but the problem seems to be that the remaining tissues often tend to redistribute themselves to give a lumpy effect. To be fair, however, the handful of surgeons who practise suction curettage do point out that the treatment is meant only for a specific age-group, mainly those who are young and *not* overweight or obese but who suffer from genetic figure problems, such as the familiar 'riding breeches' bulge of the upper thigh, a large bottom, or thick ankles, that are stubborn and impossible to shift through exercise or dieting. Women or men who are overweight are most definitely not in the running for this operation (or indeed for other forms of body reduction), nor are those over the age of about forty or those of any age whose skin is not still taut, unlined, and resilient. The reason for this is obvious: by removing surplus flesh you deprive the upper layers of skin of their natural cushioning — in much the same way as dieting — so that they must settle over new, less rounded dimensions. If the skin is slack, loose, crêpey or droopy, it will look even worse not better if the underlying supportive flesh is reduced. Aftercare, stress surgeons, also determines the final outcome. In order to avoid the formation of ripples, dimples and ridges, patients must undergo regular massage treatment for a few weeks to help the tissue to settle down smoothly and redistribute evenly; even so, post-operative lumpiness takes three or more months to disappear completely. The best results so far are reported in the reduction of a hitherto quite untreatable problem — thick ankles. In this area suction curettage works remarkably well, since there is less fat to be removed and a far more neatly circumscribed area to treat. But make no mistake, be it ankles or thighs, suction curretage is extremely uncomfortable. Inability to sit comfortably and soreness of the buttocks and even ankles lasts for a week or more, and there is extensive bruising and swelling. The ankles take the longest time of all to return to normal size and settle into their new dimensions. Sometimes surgeons advise a two-part operation to prevent causing operative trauma to the body. Treatment costs from £800 to £1500, depending on the extent and area of reduction.

The Infrastructure

The ideal candidate for cosmetic surgery should have a good bone structure. But what if this sub-structure lacks aesthetic proportion? Improving dimensions and definitions through remoulding and remodelling the nose, and building up the chin and the cheek-bones to make them appear more prominent and give them better definition, is also an inherent part of the cosmetic surgeon's job. Probably the most popular facial operation undergone by both men and women is the 'nose job' (rhinoplasty). Improvements are carried out entirely from within the nose so there is no scarring, and this often involves breaking the bone and resetting it to remove bumps and unattractive angles, carving away excess bulbous tissue, and chiselling bone and cartilage to achieve the desired refinements and new angles. Hospital stay is two to three days and a plaster cast remains over the nose for about a week. The new nose takes about six to twelve months to settle into shape, and there is considerable bruising and swelling around the eyes for a few days. The cost is about £900. Sticklers for small detail may wish to return and have tiny bits of scar tissue removed or a section of cartilage remoulded, once they have seen the final true effect unmasked by any vestige of swelling.

Implants for cheek-bones are made from silicone and are inserted either through the mouth via the inner lining of the cheek where it joins the upper gum, or, if patients are having their lower eyelids tightened or debagged, through the incision beneath the eye. Chin implants to make a receding chin more prominent, give a more attractive profile and greater definition to the face, are popped in through the mouth at the base of the lower gum or under the chin itself. Chin or cheek-bone implants run at about £750.

Facial architecture

Correcting isolated imperfections and structural defects is an accepted part of any cosmetic surgeon's job. But what if a patient's whole face leaves not one or two but a multitude of positive attributes to be desired? Is a facial jigsaw merely a wishing game for optimists? According to today's facial architects the answer is definitely no. While so-called draping methods of all soft tissue with the exception of the nose job remain firmly in the realm of the plastic surgeon, there is a whole spectrum of facial improvements that can be effected through a more adventurous and spectacular means — maxillofacial surgery, a highly evolved and skilled technique that originated in Switzerland and Austria as an offshoot of orthodontics and dentistry and involves rearranging the bones of the face. The maxillofacial area comprises the mandible (lower jaw), maxilla (upper teeth to bridge of nose), and malr (cheek-bones and the nose itself).

While the technique has been used chiefly to reconstruct the faces of war and road accident victims, surgeons such as Professor Hugo Obwegeser of Zurich and Dr Stanley Behrman of New York have devoted much pioneer work in recent years to correcting genetic defects in young people in particular, where unattractive features can cause severe psychological trauma and where the misuse of groups of facial muscles working to compensate for skeletal defects builds up chronic tension and stress which may affect a person's whole body and general health. It has been estimated that there are over fifteen million people in the USA alone with jaw deformities that cause problems with eating, chewing, speaking, and swallowing. Related bad habits create a compensatory armouring early in childhood. Commonly provoked through an uneven or open bite, childhood illnesses like juvenile rheumatoid arthritis or distrophy of muscle, bone or cartilage may cause the defect itself. 'For years this type of work was used on wounded people, but why wait until someone has a car accident to correct their faces? The suffering of some poor girl or boy with a sullen expression that masks their true character can cause deep emotional scarring', reasons Dr Behrman, who is one of America's leading facial architects, often working with a team of eight or ten people including a speech therapist, cosmetic surgeon, dentist, psychiatrist, physiotherapist, and a geneticist, to determine the child's growth-spurts and assess true bone age. The segmental procedures are planned ahead of time, and the moves strategically worked out with photos, drawings, models, casts, and plastic wedges. There are no two identical faces according to Dr Behrman, who maintains that his team is able to offer someone an option of five or six faces.

Adults who undergo surgery for mainly aesthetic rather than corrective reasons take home a wax or clay cast of their face on which they can then modify the features with putty, adding high cheek-bones, a bolder jaw line, etc. It seems that the bony complexes — a sort of facial Meccano — will bear any amount of refitting, and thus the surgical possibilities are infinite. The jaw can be brought forward to make it longer, backwards to make it shorter, down to lengthen the face and up to shorten it; augmented with a wedge to fill out a receding chin; the chin can be repositioned; the jaw box may be split, a part removed, teeth extracted, and the jaw moved back until upper and lower jaw are equal. Fractured bones are held together until healed with wires, pins and screws. In cases where the upper jaw and teeth protrude to give a Dracula effect, the sinuses, septum, and wedges of bone are cut, separated and reassembled, wired to the bony structure around the rim of the eye. The structural permutations are endless. The ingenuities of surgery ensure optimum function and the most aesthetic and harmonious appearance with the least amount of trauma. Dr Behrman is graphic — the mid-third of the face including the upper jaw, he says, is basically like putty and built to collapse like a shelf on impact to protect the brain from severe damage. The middle section goes in like a concertina. There are special disimpactive forceps used via the nose and mouth to pull it all back out. As that is the section that gives the face its proportion, rearranging these bones is an important part of the construction work. The lower jaw, on the other hand, is a hinge and as such can easily be reconstructed to work properly and look good. Not surprisingly, maxillofacial surgery is a highly costly procedure and one that in Britain as well as America will only be undertaken in cases where physical disfigurement is seen to cause both psychological and physiological problems in the individual.

Scars

The sleight of hand which is the signature of a great surgeon is reflected not only in his craftsmanship as a sculptor of bone and tissue but also in the amount of scarring — if any — that results in the process. Some surgeons' reputations are indeed made, or on the contrary ruined, by their ability or inability to leave no more than a fine, faint, infinitesimal trace of the original incision lines; others still have become renowned for their skill in repairing 'botch-ups', unsightly, red, jagged, ragged or ugly, bumpy keloid scars created by other more fumble-fisted surgeons. Scar 'therapy' usually involves opening up of the original incision and resuturing the edges more neatly together again with less tensions, finer stitches, the use of tape to press and flatten the tissues down, and possibly some fancy stitchwork such as rejoining the edges of the incision in a zigzag instead of a straight line better to follow skin tension and make the scar flatter and less conspicuous.

Although skin resurfacing techniques such as dermabrasion may remove superficial scars and minimise deeper ones, especially if they are shallow and have smooth rounded edges, acne scars or chicken-pox scars that have sharp edges, are pitted or resemble ice-pick marks or craters can only be successfully treated by such measures as miniscule skin grafts, injections of minute droplets of silicone, biopsy punches (excision) and suturing, or graft tissue replacement to pull the depressed area of skin together followed by either dermabrasion or electro-desiccation to level out the skin surface. A corticosteroid solution injected into hard raised keloid scars reduces collagen-bunching, and working in the opposite way to silicone injections, shrinks the tissues down to normal thickness.

CHAPTER 13

A Sybarite's A–Z

Whether you regard massage, facials and other salon treatments as a regular if costly necessity to help you feel and look your very best, or a delicious, sinfully sybaritic, occasional indulgence, it helps to know *what* you are getting for your money. Rip-offs abound in what has become a consumer jungle and, especially to the uninitiated, it is often the devil's own work to determine the true worth and track record of the plethora of esoteric health-beauty therapies purporting to help keep faces and bodies looking younger, smoother, softer, and sleeker. So what is the bottom line on the most popular, well tried and tested treats and treatments of the 1980s?

Aromatherapy

This has been described as the 'Rolls Royce' of beauty treatments. The sybaritic element and aura of mystique that clings to aromatherapy, originally pioneered in France and Austria in the 1940s and 50s, hinges on those eponymous plant oils whose aroma permeates the clinics of such doyennes as Michelene Arcier and Danielle Ryman. The essential oils extracted from a multitude of flowers, herbs, fruit, bark, and resins, all with their own potent and specific healing properties, are concentrated and highly volatile, supposedly penetrating through the skin into the bloodstream within minutes (research shows that lavender oil rubbed onto the skin of a guinea pig shows up in its urine twenty minutes later) and affecting the mind and emotions via inhalation and stimulus of the olfactory nerve centres. Essential oils applied in combination with deep relaxing massage combining the best elements of eastern-style acupressure, shiatsu techniques and the kneading, stroking movements of Swedish massage are used as much to treat nervous and stress-related disorders like depression, headaches, anxiety insomnia, pre-menstrual tension, fatigue, chronic sinus and bronchial congestion, as for a wide range of facial and aesthetic problems like fluid retention, cellulite, dehydrated and prematurely ageing skin, acne and related greasy skin conditions. Though it may seem incongruous and a contradiction in terms to treat oil with oil, essential oils are absorbed rapidly, leaving their 'active principles' to act therapeutically on even very greasy skin. In the case of facial skin problems, aromatherapy massage is generally combined with the application of poultices, surface peeling agents, and masks. In very rare cases does allergy occur, though people with very sensitive skin are advised to undergo a patch test prior to treatment. Severe skin irritation, rashes or burning may in fact be an indication that the oils are not 100 per cent pure. Synthetic or chemically 'doctored' oils, increasingly used by unscrupulous practictioners out to capitalise on the growing popularity of aromotherapy and other natural therapies, are not only of no benefit in treating problems of the psyche or skin but may even prove positively harmful. That is why authentic bona-fide aromatherapy doesn't come cheap — pure plant oils *are* costly to manufacture — so be prepared to pay anything from £15 to £30 for a one to one and a half hour face and body treatment.

Cathiodermie

This is today widely recognised as the first heavy-duty deep-cleansing technique which retexturises those pores and parts of the skin other treatments cannot reach. Ideal for anyone with acne-prone, spotty, coarse-pored or greasy skin, or a dry complexion that looks dull, dingy and generally lack lustre through scant regard for proper cleansing. Treatment incorporates massage with tiny rollers activated with differing frequencies of a mild galvanic current which causes light perspiration and helps to open the pores, release accumulated, deeply-embedded grime, grease and debris, and dead cells, unclogs blocked follicles, and all in all does a heavy-duty cleansing job. Part two of the treatment uses further electrical stimulus to create a layer of ozone which is absorbed into the skin, deep cleansing the pores even further, stimulating the circulation, and refining and buffing the skin's surface. Finally, conditioning liquid is massaged into the skin, and a mask is applied to further tighten, smooth and tone.

Cathiodermie generally leaves the skin looking as fresh, glowing, pink and clear as it would after a holiday in the clear Alpine air or by the seaside. It can also act as a catalyst by unplugging clogged pores, eliminating stored toxins and sebum, 'roughing up' the complexion and making it appear blotchy and freshly scrubbed for a day or two until the skin settles down. The greasier, more neglected and acne-prone skin, the more it benefits from regular and frequent cathiodermie treatments, though once or twice a month provides ideal maintenance for most skin types. Unlike many more aggressive, abrasive, deep-cleanse and surface cleaning treatments, which can dry out the skin with harsh astringents and chemical products, cathiodermie renews surface skin without risk of dehydration or damage and the regenerative effect can be as dramatic on young spotty skin as on an older, prematurely ageing or neglected one.

Electrolysis or Diathermy

Can be used either to remove superfluous hair on the face or body or to fade broken red veins. An electrical current is passed through a very fine needle, either deep into the hair follicle to destroy the root of the hair, or else inserted into the vein to cauterise the rupture and coagulate the blood. Broken veins generally need an average of two treatments each until they are sealed off, and similarly excess hair, especially if growth is particularly coarse or the follicle is damaged or curved, may need a number of treatments before it disappears permanently. Treatment may be mildly uncomfortable though it is never painful, and in the hands of a skilled operator the risk of scarring is virtually non-existent. Although it is a fallacy to believe you can emerge from an electrolysis session, especially if it is a facial treatment, say, of the upper lip or chin, without a certain degree of swelling and redness which lasts a few hours, and perhaps even some minor temporary inflammation and crusting over where the needle has pierced the skin. There is a small risk of bacterial infection after electrolysis and so the skin must be kept dry and clean; surgical spirit is the best aid to keep at hand if infection does occur. Beware of the over-zealous therapist who tries to remove too many hairs at one go; skin traumatisation is an inevitable outcome.

Electrolysis requires strict hygiene, especially since new, tighter legislation on skin piercing was passed in 1982, and a high level of training and practical skills is absolutely vital in a practitioner, so always make sure you attend a reputable salon and that the therapist is a registered member of the British Association of Electrolysis. As with ear piercing, acupuncture and tattooing, there is a potential risk not only of skin infection but of more serious hazards like herpes, AIDS and hepatitis being passed on through infected needles. In order to obtain a licence from the local health authorities, any beauty therapists practising electrolysis must prove that they have standard sterilising equipment or preferably use disposable, pre-sterilised needles — according to Dr Norman Noah of the Communicable Disease Surveillance Centre, a safer bet altogether for all forms of electrolysis.

Depilex is a more recent electronic tweezer method of hair removal, which is generally received with thumbs down from beauty therapists in general, although certain beauticians claim the method works well for those people with very fine or minimal hair growth.

Electromagnetic Therapy

This was first developed over twelve years ago when it was discovered that astronauts who had been beyond the earth's magnetic field had lost calcium from their bones, a disorder that responded quickly and well to this treatment. There is increasing scientific evidence that electrical energy can accelerate the healing of bone fractures, torn muscles, and ligaments by as much as 40 to 50 per cent, so not surprisingly pulse high frequency (PHF) is used both in hospitals as well as by physiotherapist, osteopaths, and even vets in the case of racehorses etc, as well as by certain specialised health/beauty clinics as back-up therapy for an ever-growing number of injuries and post-operative conditions. Treatment is simple and painless and is given via a machine that emits short bursts of high-frequency radio waves which create a 'magnetic field' over the damaged area. The pulsating effect causes heat to be dissipated within the tissues, gently stimulating cellular metabolism (i.e. anabolism) and so speeding up the body's self-repair mechanism. Energy penetrates the tissues by up to eight to ten inches, working equally well through clothing, plastercasts, and surgical dressings. Reports suggest that PHF 'mends' skin as efficiently as bone or internal organs and as such it is used to treat bones, wounds, and ulcers, to speed and improve healing of cosmetic surgery, in particular to prevent swelling, haematoma (bleeding), and bruising, and to minimise the risk of keloid or ordinary scar tissue formation. Whatever the condition and area being treated, PHF is almost always used routinely over the liver and adrenal glands to stimulate further the body's entire metabolism and healing processes, while generally calming the central nervous system — especially beneficial after severe injury, shock or surgery. The number of treatments varies according to the condition, and the cost of one 30–45-minute session may be between £10–£15. Some clinics rent out small portable PHF units for home use, an effort and money-saver if you are in the running for half a dozen treatments or more.

Laser Therapy

Revolutionary breakthrough treatments and products in the world of beauty are rarely as innovative or as original as their proponents would have us believe. Consumer expectations and fickleness being what they are, flagging long-term popularity invariably casts shadows on the early days of heady hype and hollow promises. For evidence of this example of Newton's law, one need look no further than the much vaunted cold beam laser 'face-lift', the 'hottest' rejuvenating story of the early 80s, a hodgepodge of all the best elements of serious medicine, space-age technology, and natural holistic therapy, combined in a bid for ever, or at least longer, lasting youth.

Introduced to Britain in 1981, treatment consists of passing a 'cold' laser beam over the facial acupuncture points (shades of cosmetic acupuncture a treatment which enjoyed brief popularity in the late '70s) and areas of lined, wrinkled, crêpey skin to stimulate and shock skin tissues into renewing itself more effectively, while simultaneously 'mending' already worn and ageing skin. Cosmetic benefits — tighter, brighter, less lined skin — are based on the premise, virtually identical to that used in facial acupuncture, that the laser stimulates the flow of blood, tones the muscles, and acts as a catalyst for cell renewal. Yet there is, as with facial acupuncture, very little real evidence to support the claims that the cold beam laser — according to many doctors no stronger than a 100-watt light bulb — can affect the activity of skin cells or in any way alter and affect the nature of skin tissue. Many British doctors in fact have dismissed the treatment as a con and about as effective as shining a battery-charged torchlight over the skin. Limited, ill-documented research, carried out at amongst other places the Korvin Otto Hospital in Budapest on laboratory animals, has shown that when damaged tissues are treated with a laser, healing is more rapid and complete than when left to recover naturally, and other Swedish studies have shown that damaged muscles can be healed and strengthened more effectively through laser treatment. But damaged skin gears up its renewal system remarkably effectively at the best of times, and whether laser energy is actually responsible for prompting fibroblast cells to lay down new collagen or repairing damaged collagen and elastin remains extremely dubious. Treatment seems to work best on relatively healthy skin, as yet unravaged by the onslaught of time, stress, illness, and neglect. Women and men in their thirties, forties and early fifties, who have undergone laser facials as a preventive measure against premature ageing in much the same way as they might invest in facials to maintain a smooth complexion, have reported that most favourable results include a softening of nose-to-mouth lines, the easing of lines of tightness and tiredness caused through muscular strain, and the smoothing of slack, puffy tissues around the lower eyelids. But does it last? Not long enough, given the cost.

Initial results are probably due to the mildly irritant effect the treatment has on the skin, causing the very top layer of skin to swell up almost imperceptibly in response to treatment, a perfectly normal reaction that occurs during most types of friction, massage, etc. Existing lines and grooves will, plumped up by the slightly swollen skin tissues, appear less deeply defined, but the effect is alas short-lived. The second reason why effects seem initially encouraging is due to the cleansing routine and use of serums after the laser treatment, which have a brightening and tightening effect on the tissues. In essence, laser treatment provides a superb, relaxing, first-class facial and the accompanying results that you'd expect, but the outlay can be hefty, £15–£25 per session, and most therapists, if they are honest, report a dramatic falling off in the number of new or second-time-round clients asking for laser therapy. Dr Paul Salmon, President of the European Laser Association, is particularly concerned about the risk of eye injury, an inherent danger with all lasers, even the low-powered cold beam variety used by beauticians. Lasers used by the beauty trade *do* vary in strength, ranging from the Class I, II or III machines whose power is extremely low — perhaps 1 or 2 milliwatts — to the more powerful Class 3B equipment which has both a higher milliwattage and a more deeply penetrating frequency or wavelength. Disconcerting too are reports filtering through of 'cowboy' doctors who have set themselves up as specialised 'laser dermatologists', treating all variety of skin ailments from verrucas to wrinkles with the use of more powerful surgical lasers, such as the carbon dioxide laser. In expert hands these are perfectly safe for the treatment of warts, verrucas, skin tags and other lesions, but on no account should a powerful surgical laser *ever* be used on facial skin tissue to 'burn away' wrinkles and lines: the result of burning and scarring could be permanent and horrifically unsightly.

Massage

The skin is the primary transmitter of the myriad messages and impulses received by the muscles, joints, nerve cells, capillaries, glands, and internal organs. Therefore the all-important intuitive relationship of trust, empathy and silent communication, or indeed its opposite, discord and tension, begins from the very first moment a masseur or masseuse lays their hands on your skin. Through touch, skin gives you your very first emotional, physical and psychic feedback, which, if we're honest, usually can and should instinctively be trusted. A good massage, apart from all its far-reaching physical benefits, helps to rekindle and cultivate jaded tactile senses and enhance body awareness. It leaves the skin not only looking radiant, refined and softened but tunes up its finer surface sensations, making you feel more alive and responsive to tactile stimuli. Every first-class facial, apart from routine deep-cleansing, surface exfoliation, the elimination of blackheads and whiteheads, the use of masks and an application of conditioning and regenerating products, includes a few minutes or more of face and neck massage to relax the muscles, ease out lines of fatigue and tension, improve the circulation, warm the tissues, and help skincare products penetrate the skin more effectively. Top therapists who really know their job are sensitive to the degree of stress, tension and tiredness in their clients, will often massage the neck and shoulders and upper back, which diffuses stored tension and stimulates the flow of blood to the facial tissues. Some may even message the scalp and feet to ease tight muscles. Puffy cheek tissues and bags under the eyes which are often the direct result of sinus congestion, fluid retention and inflammation, respond often dramatically well to neuromuscular massage, incorporating firm thumb and finger acupressure, applied to the acupuncture points along the eyebrows and sides of the nose, on the temples, inner eye, and along the rim of the cheekbones and eye-sockets, all directly linked and corresponding to the sinus cavities.

When it comes to more intensive, specialised forms of massage, finding a good practitioner isn't always straightforward or an easy matter. One often tends to discover the finest masseurs by chance, through word of mouth passed on by the true cognoscenti of body massage, such as dancers, athletes, actors, other therapists, in short anyone who has a highly developed sense of physical-cum-psychological well-being. But like idyllic holiday retreats, gourmet recipes and restaurants, the identity and whereabouts of these favourite doyennes of massage can remain a jealously guarded secret, devilishly hard to elicit from even one's closest friends, which is why I have included my own list of tried and tested top face and body therapists at the back of this book. In addition to the low profile kept by its practitioners, the massage itself comes in many seemingly weird and wonderful esoteric forms, and trying to work out what type of treatment is best suited to your individual needs, how it works, and what kind of track record it enjoys in the field of beauty and holistic therapy, remains a perpetual challenge to novice and old hand alike. Although aromatherapy massage is undoubtedly the finest massage to combine surface aesthetics with inner therapy, shiatsu (Japanese finger pressure or acupressure — acupuncture without the needles), which relies principally on intensive finger and thumb pressure exerted slowly in concentration over virtually every square inch of the body, can put you in possession of the nearest thing to a new body you are likely to get, while connective tissue massage with its emphasis on activating lymphatic drainage can greatly help women suffering from cellulite and fluid retention.

Mesotherapy

This is a relatively new therapy that hails from France, where certain GPs and therapists are claiming considerable success in the treatment of chronic pain and nervous ailments as well as localised figure problems — cellulite in particular. The rationale behind mesotherapy (from the Greek 'meso' meaning small) is a sound and relatively convincing one, in theory at any rate. Treat target trouble spots directly by giving only very small doses of medicine via localised 'micro' injections, and you should get to the root of the trouble faster and with less risk of such side effects as digestive upsets, delayed or incomplete absorption, nausea, drowsiness, and the addiction often inherent in giving drugs orally or intravenously. Developed during the '50s, mesotherapy is now practised by over 5000 doctors in pain clinics and hospitals throughout France, Italy and Germany. The drugs used may be either mainstream medical — analgesics, anti-inflammatory, antibiotics, etc — or homoeopathic, plant-based extracts, vitamins, minerals, and enzymes.

Sports injuries, arthritis, back pain, neuralgia, tennis elbow, migraine, muscle, joint or tendon disorders respond particularly well to mesotherapy, as does any condition, like cellulite, related to faulty circulation or fluid retention, which may be treated with vascodilating substances and drugs that resemble thyroid extracts aimed at helping to speed up safely the rate of metabolism. When it comes to reducing stubborn surplus fat that doesn't respond to dieting, some doctors have been known virtually to guarantee slimmer hips and thighs after fifteen 10-minute sessions, with the odd booster needed to maintain the improvement. Well-worn claims, it is true, but even though a new import to this country, mesotherapy does have its growing number of advocates who have emerged more streamlined after a course of treatment.

The tools of treatment are, however, quaint, even bordering on the bizarre. Surplus fat may be attacked, for example, with the 'hedgehog' or multi-injector, an 8,12 or even 16-needle syringe designed to treat larger areas such as thighs and bottom. Sensation varies and depends a lot on individual padding and pain thresholds, but discomfort can be minimised by the incorporation of a local anaesthetic into the mixture to dull the sting. More recent and altogether high-tech is the Pistormatic, an electronic staple-gun syringe which rests on a moveable cradle and is electronically programmed to shoot backwards and forwards to give either an intermittent or rapid series of injections, releasing varying doses of serum with bullseye staccato precision. Treatment costs around £12 to £15 per session.

CHAPTER 14

Looking Ahead — A.D. 2000 and Beyond

'There is no field of preventive medicine more optimistic than dermatology.' Sanguine sentiments surely from Dr Albert Kligman of the University of Pennsylvania Medical School, which, based as they are rather less on fanciful conjecture and hypotheses than on hard scientific evidence, should inspire hope in the heart of anyone concerned about the future of their own as well as their children's and grandchildren's skin.

Dr Kligman's optimism illustrates the immense inroads made recently in the control, treatment and prevention of skin disorders, developments in methods of diagnosis and treatment that, as he sees it, will continue to grow as dermatology increasingly embraces the latest high-tech wizardry and incorporates facets of the 'new age' sciences such as molecular biology, genetic engineering, bio-engineering, and chemotherapy. As the average human lifespan continually extends itself by another notch or two, more and more of us are concerned not only about preserving the quality of our life and health during the extra years and decades allotted to us but also about maintaining our looks into the bargain. The whole concept of ageing 'gracefully' — too often a euphemism for following the line of least resistance to invasion by warts, wrinkles, grey hair, flab and all — has become anathema to many of us as we approach the twenty-first century. If that deadly term 'middle age' seems increasingly a quaint, meaningless, label destined for obsolescence — how *do* you after all distinguish nowadays between a fit, healthy, active and attractive so-called middle aged 38- or 45-year old and a relative 'youngster' of twenty-five? — so the more emotive words 'elderly' and 'old', which chillingly conjure up a spectre of impending senility, are themselves rapidly becoming devalued

as the common coinage used to describe fit, energetic, productive, attractive men and women whose chronological age just
happens to add up to sixty or even seventy-plus.

Women, whose average lifespan is now nudging eighty and
rising, obviously will continue to have a vested interest in
remaining not only young in spirit but in looks for longer —
which, according to Dr Kligman, they can. 'Any woman can and
should look great at eight-five. There is no need to have one
blotch, one skin-cancer lesion, sags, creases, or bags. Certainly as
we age, we all develop certain wrinkles and lines; how many and
where they form is determined by one's genetic inheritance. But
they need not be too many or too ageing.'

Dr Kligman forsees a time when the realisation of just how
deeply damaging and ageing are the effects of the entire UV light
spectrum will finally sink in, to most of us, and wearing cosmetics
and skin creams with in-built UVA+B sunscreens all the year
round will become routine skin care. Since he firmly believes that
heat is almost as damaging to skin as UV light because it
potentiates the effects of those rays, pigments which reflect IR
(infra-red) will be, he hopes, eventually discovered and synthesised, to be incorporated into the new 'therapeutic' cosmetics
of the future. Blushers, foundation, powder, eyeshadow, lip
stick, based on revolutionary protective formulae that screen out
all forms of radiation could well lend an entire new aspect to
'putting on a face' in the year 2000. The idea doesn't seem unduly
improbable if you follow some of the clues offered by nature.

Put a naked man or woman in the bottom of the Grand Canyon
and they're dead in about an hour, yet frogs can sit out there
endlessly, protected from hypothermia, dehydration, and burning by crystalline reflector cells in their skin. There are certain
species of birds in the Sahara Desert that lay their eggs in the sun
without the risk of them ending up hardboiled. Why? One of the
scientists' greatest challenges lies in discovering similar pigments
for use in products that will protect human skin in a similar
fashion. So, although twenty-first-century cosmetics may look no
different from their present-day counterparts, what they may do
is offer a hitherto unimaginable trump card in preserving the
youth and beauty of underlying skin, thus redefining the entire
'glamour only' principle of cosmetics as we recognise it today.

New Age Cosmetics

Similarly, dermatologists like Dr Kligman have tremendous faith in the cosmetic use and rejuvenating potential of such potent drugs as vitamin A acid, a derivative of retinoic acid (synthetic vitamin-A derivatives) used nowadays successfully to treat severe acne, psoriasis and chronic congenital skin diseases, and a substance called 5-Fluorouracil, which is sometimes prescribed for cancerous or pre-cancerous skin growths. Both substances systematically destroy skin cells through a chemical action which weakens the bonds between cells, so loosening and eliminating tissue that has become damaged or mutated. When used as anti-cancer, anti-acne or psoriasis treatment, this severely 'roughs up' the skin, burning, blistering, and crusting over its surface and involving weeks or months of sometimes gross traumatisation which eventually allows the upper skin to shed itself and reveal a new, healthier, smooth surface free of blotches, sunspots, and roughness. The aesthetic clincher: a reduction and softening or plumping up of lines and wrinkles, marked tightening (as is the case following dermabrasion which tightens the skin by 10–20 per cent) of the epidermis, improved supply of blood to the tissues, accelerated cell renewal and, most significant of all, increased fibroblast cell activity which results in the laying down of new supplies of fresh, young collagen fibres within the dermis. Most doctors remain understandably cautious in the extreme regarding the use of vitamin A acid or 5-F for anything other than serious or life-threatening skin problems. But Dr Kligman speculates that in decades to come, the best skin-care creams could well contain substances such as vitamin A acid in very low concentrations sufficient either to repair sun-ravaged skin or maintain healthy skin as it ages by nudging the activity of fibroblast and basal cells and blood supply. At his Ageing Skin Clinic at the University of Pennsylvania Medical School, Dr Kligman has observed what he terms 'fantastic effects' as an aesthetic offshoot of vitamin-A-acid-therapy on older patients with damaged skin. Histological studies (examining tiny sections of live skin tissue under the microscope) show that the substance, taken internally or applied externally, hastens the skin's renewal and repair processes, accelerating collagen synthesis, cell division, and the flow of blood. 'I'm sure that in the future people with prematurely ageing, sun-damaged skin will be able to bring their face and other areas of skin under control with a bout of intensive vitamin-A acid-therapy, then go onto a low maintenance dose.' But vitamin A acid, like 5-F, is a potent substance aimed at wounding the skin, which is why it works in controlling serious disorders in the first place. The challenge remains to reach an optimal dose at which beneficial results are achieved without damage — irritation, burning, stinging, dryness — a particular problem with a fair skin which, of course, is the very skin type most likely to suffer cumulative sun damage and therefore the likeliest contender for this type of therapy, were it ever to become a commercially viable proposition.

Stalling Mechanisms

Other than the obvious, quantifiable, degenerative effects of sunlight and general weathering, scientists remain stumped as to why skin, or indeed any other part of the body, finally cracks up at any given age. Taking into account the existence of an in-built, genetic 'time clock', a theory long subscribed to by many scientists, the likeliest explanation is that tissue cells are simply programmed to go slow at a certain point in a person's life, becoming 'senile' and finally packing up altogether. According to some biochemists, the faltering rate and impaired quality of cell production may well be dictated by the ebb and decline in production of certain, as yet unidentified, 'growth factors', hormone-like substances which turn on the growth mechanism within the fibroblasts, the master cells of the dermis principally responsible for manufacturing collagen, mucopolysaccharides, and other constituents of the tissues. In vitro (i.e. test tube) studies show that, for example, the turnover of dermal cells can be increased by adding fetal calf serum, a tissue serum taken from animals. By identifying and isolating similar growth proteins in human tissue and finding ways in which to modulate or regulate their production within the fibroblast cells, scientists reason that it may one day prove possible to maintain a steady turnover of young healthy skin tissue well into the last decades of a person's life — yet another example of the hopes genetic engineering may hold in store for future youth and beauty-conscious generations.

Dr Norman Orentreich, clinical Associate Professor of Dermatology at New York University School of Medicine, is following his own hunches in attempting to trace the hormonal and endocrinological clues to ageing. He is currently researching a 'blood washing' technique called plasmapheresis — a lengthy and costly procedure not without some minor risks — in the hopes that this may modify the rate and nature of the ageing process. By cleansing the blood through eliminating and replacing fresh quantities of its fluid component, plasma, Dr Orentreich observes that those substances in the blood which contribute to the slowdown of cell division might be eradicated and the action of other substances which enhance cell metabolism strengthened. It is all very much in the early experimental stages and pretty much a long shot at that, but it isn't totally impossible that plasmapheresis may one day yield a secret or two worth knowing about the factors which hasten our physical decline.

The Light Fantastic

Already harnessed in ever-expanding, diverse fields of medicine, laser technology seems poised to revolutionise the day-to-day *modus operandi* of the twenty-first century skin specialist in a most spectacular manner. It is surely no exaggeration to describe the laser beam as a space-age supertool, a magic wand with a broad gamut of functions in realms as diverse as transport, communications, beauty, defence, genetic engineering, entertainment, space travel, and mining.

Once familiar to us only as the deadly exterminating ray wielded by the likes of James Bond, Flash Gordon, and the wagers of Star Wars, the imprint of the laser, a mere twenty years after its inception, can be witnessed as much in the mundane and day-to-day as in the scientifically way-out. The holes in razor blades and the teats of baby-feed bottles are punched by laser, as are the invisible perforations in cigarette paper; Buzz Aldrin beamed one off the moon and bounced it back off earth to gauge the distance between the two planets, yet, more prosaically, the laser also makes light work of dissolving dental fillings, aligning subway tunnels, keeping stock at the supermarket checkout, rejuvenating the skin, or creating holograms, three-dimensional 'light' pictures which are totally lifelike until you walk right through them.

But nowhere are the possibilities of the laser 'knife' more infinite or potentially revolutionary than in the field of medicine, where sci-fi's deadliest deterrent has been harnessed by surgeons to prolong and even save lives, streamlining and simplifying standard surgical procedures, and inspiring innovative treatments unthinkable within the limits of conventional surgery.

So just how does it all work? The word laser stands for Light Amplification by Stimulated Emission of Radiation, a fascinating process originally predicted by Einstein back in 1917 that involves bombarding a basic substance such as gas, liquid, crystal or other solid matter with light, which is then repeatedly reflected off a series of mirrored panels, multiplying the original power hundreds or thousands of times over. The result? A narrow concentrated beam of light which can be converted into heat intense enough to drill a hole in a diamond, slice through steel, bone and concrete, or provide just enough power to lift the type clean off this page without so much as marking the paper.

The key to this power and precision lies in the laser's near magical quality — coherence. Quite simply, unlike ordinary diffuse or reflected light, which is made up of a scattering of different and randomly shifting wavelengths (i.e. colours), laser light is composed of just one single frequency, its light waves perfectly aligned in tight parallel lines or bundles which move forward 'in phase', that is, in a narrow, consistently straight beam and in one direction only.

Put graphically, the laser beam is to ordinary light what a chaotic mob is to a well drilled army, whose columns of soliders advance shoulder to shoulder in unison, swiftly and selectively destroying their target while the rabble run helter skelter creating random destruction. It is this neat uniformity of the light pattern which makes, say, an 8 watt Argon laser capable of generating energy one thousand times stronger than the power of the sun (it is also, by the way, 80,000 times stronger than the cold beam lasers used by beauticians), its beam so minutely focused that it can pinpoint one single blood cell and punch seven holes in it!

Into the Infinite

Since laser light must first be absorbed in order to produce the heat which destroys tissues, its different uses in medicine are largely dictated by the various wavelengths produced. For instance, the blue-green beam of the Argon laser passes straight through unpigmented tissue and is absorbed by melanin and haemoglobin (red blood cells), so it is ideal for cauterising ruptured blood vessels, controlling bleeding tumours, bleaching port wine stains and certain tattoos, or punching a hole in the iris of someone suffering from glaucoma. The Neodymium Yag infra-red laser is more powerful still, and will stem very deep-seated bleeding, pulverise kidney stones or destroy certain cancers, but since its beam is invisible, it must first be mounted on a helium-neon 'aiming beam' — identical to those used in the beauty trade — in order to spotlight the exact target to be treated. The mighty carbon dioxide laser 'knife' also emits an invisible beam which is absorbed by all tissues — the absorbed energy is converted into heat which vaporises the tissues, irrespective of their colour, and it is therefore increasingly used to replace the scalpel and slice through tissues at over 100° C.

Such phenomenal blasting power would of course prove unthinkably dangerous were it not for the fail safe that allows surgeons to 'pulse' the energy by programming a laser to fire a precise given strength for perhaps no more than half a second at a time. The difference between applying enough energy to seal a blood vessel or blasting a hole through someone's stomach depends on a matter of a millisecond. And indeed, overkill is a very real risk of laser therapy when applied to skin: as with any other method of surface skin destruction such as dermabrasion or cryotherapy, the laser *will* produce scarring if tissues are destroyed at levels over 2/10ths of a millimetre deep.

But provided you get your timing right — and surgeons emphasise that laser work does require extra mechanical skills as well as a steady hand and eagle-eye — the laser knife scores over the scalpel and chemicals in its speed and finesse, the ultimate in surgical elegance. By exerting the utmost control and spot-on timing it is possible to cut, vaporise and seal off human tissue with only a fraction of the time and trauma involved in conventional surgery. The advantages of the laser include its ability to seal promptly blood vessels, lymphatic nerve endings and coagulate blood as it cuts into tissue, eliminating heavy bleeding and therefore all related complications. It automatically also sterilises the tissues, minimising the risk of infection and, being painless, it requires no general anaesthetic. Since there is no incision, stitches and scar tissue are a thing of the past in laser skin surgery and, more important still, the laser's bullseye focusing power means only affected cells and tissues are treated without the risk of damage to healthy surrounding skin.

Its use in dermatology is expanding constantly. Dermatologists, plastic surgeons and ear, nose, and throat specialists have adopted lasers with particular gusto, and it isn't hard to see why. Removing lumps, bumps, blemishes, and growths, malignant or benign, be they nodules on the vocal chords, polyps inside the mouth, nose or ear, skin tumours, verrucas, warts or haemorrhoids, becomes relative child's play with the laser. This means that surgeons working in hospitals equipped with laser technology can treat many more patients than is normally possible, because treatment takes only a few minutes, involves no anaesthetic, stitching, dressing, cleaning up, and therefore can take place in the out-patients department with minimum fuss or discomfort to the patient.

Dermabrasion, whose success to date is determined almost entirely by surgical sleight and steadiness of hand, may also one day be conducted via a combined laser-computer-scanner unit. Dermatologists at the Laser Research and Treatment Centre at New York's Albert Einstein College of Medicine have recently perfected a new 'fully automatic' computerised 'laserbrasion', which they say ensures a uniform, non-messy, bloodless, superficial skin peel that entails rather less post-operative unsightliness and discomfort than when carried out by human hand. Potential candidates would have to be screened and 'patch tested' as rigorously as those contemplating regular dermabrasion.

In Tel Aviv, plastic surgeon Dr Shamai Giler sees an average of eight patients an hour, treating conditions as diverse as skin cancers, broken veins and rhynophyma, verrucas, brown 'age' spots, genital or facial warts and herpes, seborroeic or solar keratoses, and tattoos, cutting down extensively on what would normally, as in England, be a very lengthy waiting list of patients awaiting treatment. Unlike, say, cryotherapy (liquid nitrogen 'freezing'), the depth of tissue destruction can be precisely controlled with minimum risk of scarring, and sections of 'suspect' tissue can be excised intact more easily for histological analysis to establish whether or not any cancerous changes have taken place.

Though many dermatological operations rarely constitute a matter of life or death, they do nevertheless often help make life more bearable for many men, women and children. One such area in which doctors are using the Argon laser to try and alleviate years of anguish and embarrassment is in the treatment of disfiguring port wine stains (birthmarks) by sealing off the millions of tiny leaking blood vessels which 'flood' the affected area, giving it its livid appearance. Alas, in this case — as with tattoos also, incidentally — the laser often falls far short of being a magic wand because not all birthmarks are created equal and therefore differ greatly in their response to treatment. Doctors stress that although many sufferers can be helped to regain a near-normal appearance, lengthy testing is often required to establish whether a birthmark or tattoo can be faded without the risk of burning or scarring the skin.

So far, laser treatment for skin disorders is confined either to private specialists and clinics — your GP can refer you to a suitable practitioner — or to some of the few major teaching hospitals in Britain lucky enough to be able to invest in the latest technology. For, at the cost of about £30,000 or more per laser with fibres that constantly wear out and need replacing at £250 a throw, the laser is in no imminent danger of making the scalpel redundant, and unless you happen to be admitted to a hospital with its own laser unit, as for example University College Hospital in London, your chances of obtaining treatment on the NHS remain pretty remote at the moment. By the early 2000s, however, the cost of laser technology may well have become more competitive as has happened with videos, bringing down market prices and making treatment a more viable cost-effective proposition, readily available on demand.

Seconds

As I have outlined in earlier chapters, the complex structure and function of human skin make it a brilliantly conceived biological 'one-off', not easy to fake or replicate in synthetic form in a laboratory with a mock-up of artificial materials. However, come the next few decades, scientists may well manage to perfect a synthetic skin substitute, not nearly as hardy, realistic or durable as the real thing but nevertheless with sufficient characteristic features to provide a wide range of uses in medicine. What, for example, is desperately needed by doctors treating patients with severe life-threatening wounds and burns, whose skin has been mutilated to a degree that vital body functions are disrupted, is a temporary 'stand in' skin to cover the site of damage and prevent essential fluids from oozing out and bacteria from creeping into the body. Normally a skin graft taken from an undamaged part of the body would be used, but when a burn is widespread there may simply not be enough human skin to go round, and cadaver or animal skin is grafted; but this can only be an arbitrary stop-gap measure because, being foreign tissue, such grafts are invariably rejected by the body within 3–25 days.

Plastic surgeons are now eagerly experimenting with a variety of synthetic 'second skins' that hold tremendous potential promise for the future survival and recovery rate of burn victims. A clear polyurethane covering is being tested with a certain success in patients with relatively superficial burns, to protect damaged skin like a piece of gauze, keeping the area moist, admitting oxygen, yet repelling bacteria, while allowing new skin cells to move around freely and initiate the healing process. Although it has been found this material may speed healing, it is of no use in second or third-degree burns where the underlying blood vessels have been destroyed.

Another synthetic skin, just 1/100th inch thick, has been designed, using a compound of silicone rubber and nylon-coated chemical collagen derivatives which is proving superior to animal skin as it isn't rejected and can be stored indefinitely. But by far the most impressive-sounding piece of skin 'design' so far, soon to be marketed, hails from MIT — the Massachusetts Institute of Technology — and is a hybrid incorporating cowhide, shark cartilage, and plastic. The substitute bears an artful resemblance to the real McCoy, having two layers, an 'epidermis' made of silicone, and a 'dermis' composed of a mixture of cowhide and shark cartilage proteins, which cannily resembles human skin but cannot trigger rejection from the host tissue. The skin is manufactured via freeze-drying, vacuum treatment, baking and bonding to form a soft, pliable, porous sheet — a bit like paper kitchen towelling — which can be draped over burn sites of any depth and size. The fibres within the bottom layer trigger renewed proliferation of the patient's own collagen fibres and are eventually replaced by the new growth. The process is most ingenious: nerve fibres, blood vessels and connective tissue all grow upwards into the substitute skin which, becoming su-perfluous, gradually breaks down and disperses, to be replaced by a brand-new layer of human tissue. The outer silicone layer which acts purely as a temporary protective covering is peeled off as the healing process gets underway, to be replaced by small pieces of epidermis taken from other parts of the patient's body. Man-made skin is of course still in its infancy, and much more clinical testing is needed before it will be available for widespread use. Still on the agenda is a brief to develop a membrane which will cover burns and wounds and remain there until the patient's own skin has fully formed beneath, eliminating the need for interim epidermal grafting and patch-up procedures that involve using other sections of the patient's own skin.

Taking the Plasters

High technology is also very much in evidence in the new 'transepidermal drug delivery systems' that have recently initiated a whole new approach to drug taking. Placing a tiny plaster on your wrist or behind your ear whenever you have a headache or feel sick could well make pill-popping a thing of the past for future generations of drug users. Developed as a result of the combined research and development teams of pharmaceutical companies such as Ciba-Geigy and Alza, an American company responsible for pioneering new methods of administering drug therapy, drugs which so far are already prescribed in stick-on plaster form for slow release through the skin into the bloodstream include those to counteract nausea and motion sickness, and nitroglycerine to dilate the blood vessels and arteries of people suffering from angina and other cardiovascular disorders. The beauty of taking your medicine transepidermally is that unlike injections and oral medication, release of the drug into the bloodstream can be precisely controlled, minimising risks such as gastric upsets and other side-effects, while ensuring that concentration of the drug remains steady, and the duration of its action prolonged and enhanced without any chance of an overdose. It is certainly the neatest, no-fuss method of drug taking ever invented, and doctors predict a steady growth in the different varieties of drugs eventually available to us 'by skin' as well as in micro-implant form to be placed just beneath the skin's surface —already a common method of administering hormone replacement therapy for menopausal symptoms.

Idealised, immortalised, lauded by artists throughout the ages as the chief inspiration of love and symbol of beauty, the skin is one of the last remaining parts of the human body to retain its aura of mystique and its powerful romantic imagery, tempting us as ever to project our fantasies upon its surface. But taking into account present development as well as future prophecies, it becomes increasingly obvious that the full possibilities of human skin as a 'window' on the body as well as the scope for enhancing its condition are only only just dawning. Skin a surface issue? Far from it. From drug-delivery vehicle to psychosomatic and environmental sensor, the skin's inner depths and dimension are a constant source of enlightenment and encouragement to anyone concerned with its beauty. And that's surely each one of us, poet, lover, romantic or no. On the surface, and beneath, future prospects have never looked better.

Useful Addresses

Action Against Allergy Association, 31 Abbey Parade, Merton High Street, London SW19.

Society of Skin Camouflage, Western Pitmenzies, Auchternuchty, Fife, Scotland.

Micheline Arcier, 7 William Street, London SW1. 01–235 3545
Specialist in aromatherapy.

Association of Suntanning Operators, 32 Grayshott Road, London SW11. 01–228 6077

The Bluestone Clinic, 16 Harley House, Marylebone Road, London NW1. 01–935 7933/8958
Electromagnetic therapy, remedial massage, laser facials.

Bournemouth Centre of Natural Medicine, 26A Sea Road, Boscombe, Bournemouth. 0202 36354.

British Association of Beauty Therapists, Suite 5, Wolseley House, Oriel Road, Cheltenham, Glos GL50.

British Association of Beauty Therapy and Cosmetology, 5 Greenways, Winchcombe, Cheltenham, Glos. 0242 603243.

British Association of Dermatologists, 7 John Street, London WC1. 01–404 0092.

British Association of Electrolysysts, 16 Quakers Mede, Haddenham, Bucks HP17 8EB.

British Association of Plastic Surgeons, R.C.S., 35 Lincoln's Inn Fields, London WC2. 01–242 7750.

British Association of Therapeutical Hypnotists, 95 Prospect Road, Woodford Green, Essex. 01–505 8720.

British Biosthetic Society, 2 Birkdale Drive, Bury, Greater Manchester.

British Naturopathic and Osteopathic Association, 6 Netherall Gardens, London NW3 5RR. 01–435 8728.

British Red Cross Society, 6 Grosvenor Crescent, London SW1. 01–235 7131.

Jacqueline Burgess-Wall, The Beauty Studio, 467A Finchley Road, London N4. 01–794 4286.
Specialist in nail, hand and foot treatments.

Cathiodermie Advisory Centre, R. Robson Ltd, The Old Pound House, London Road, Sunningdale, Berks SL6 0DJ. 0990 26133.

Sally Gilbert Wilson, 136 Harley Street, London W1. 01–486 7490.
CTM massage, facial acupuncture, mesotherapy, acne treatments, Gerovital therapy.

Julie Hacker, 48 Montagu Mansions, London W1. 01–935 3424.
Acne treatments.

Helena Harnik Clinic, 19 Upper Berkeley Street, London W1. 01–724 1518.
Acne treatment and therapy for problem skins. Non-surgical peeling.

Images, 19 Paddington Street, London W1. 01–935 3166.
Cathiodermie, chua K'A massage.

Institute of Clinical Aromatherapy, 22 Bromley Road, London SE6 2TP. 01–690 2149.

Institute of Electrolysis, 251 Seymour Grove, Manchester M16 0DS. 061–881 5306.

Institute of Trichologists, 228 Stockwell Road, London SW9 9SU. 01–733 2056.

The Jean Worth Beauty Therapy Advisory and Consultation Bureau, Wildeacres, Ellesmere Road, St Georges, Weybridge, Surrey. Weybridge 42014.

Marietta Kavanagh, 4A William Street, London SW1. 01–235 4106.
Specialist in neuromuscular therapy/massage/acne treatment.

Philip Kingsley Clinic, 54 Green Street, London W1. 01–629 4004.
Hair and scalp problems.

Mandy Langford, 10 Alexander Street, London W2. 01–727 2006.
Hypnotherapy.

London and Counties Society of Physiologists, 100 Waterloo Road, Blackpool, Lancs. 0253 403548.

The London Mesotherapy Centre, 23 Wimpole Street, London W1. 01–935 5054. 37 Devonshire Place, London W1.

The Mastectomy Advisory Service, 40 Eglantine Avenue, Belfast BT9 6DX.

National Eczema Society, 27 Doyle Gardens, London NW10.

Natural Health Foundation, The Ryepeck, Thames Street, Sunbury-on-Thames, Middx. 54 84968.

The Psoriasis Association, 300 Wellingborough Road, Northampton NN1 4ED.

Register of British Acupuncturists, 94 Banstead Road South, Sutton, Surrey SM2 5LH. 01–642 4161.

Danièle Ryman, Suite 101, Park Lane Hotel, Piccadilly, London W1. 01–493 6630.
Specialist in aromatherapy and deep-cleanse/revitalising facials.

School of Herbal Medicine, 148 Forest Road, Tunbridge Wells, Kent TN2 5EY. 0892 30400.

Society of Cosmetic Chemists, 56 Kingsway, London WC2 6DX. 01–242 3800.

Strands, 62 Duke Street, London W1. 01–629 5622.
Laser and other facials.

Tisserand Aromatics Ltd (aromatherapy), 52–54 St Aubyns Road, Fishersgate, Brighton BN4 1PE. Brighton 412139.

For advice and additional information on massage and other alternative methods of healing, and natural therapies:

The Alternative Health Centre, 266 Fulham Road, London SW. 01–351 2726.
Specialists in natural therapy for psoriasis and eczema.

The Churchill Centre, 22 Montagu Street, London W1. 01–402 9475.

Community Health Foundation, 188–194 Old Street, London EC1. 01–251 4076.

Neal's Yard Therapy Rooms, 2 Neal's Yard, Covent Garden, London WC2. 01–379 7662.

Index